Unlimited Energy

Jacquelyn Lyon BS, MBA

Skyward Publishing

Dallas, Texas

Copyright 2003 by Skyward Publishing, Inc.

Publisher: Skyward Publishing, Inc
                Dallas, Texas
                Phone: 972-490-8988

                Web Site: www.skywardpublishing.com

Library of Congress Cataloging-in-Publication Data

Lyon, Jacquelyn, 1947-
  Unlimited energy / by Jacquelyn Lyon.
     p. cm.
  ISBN 1-881554-12-0
  1. Alternative medicine. 2. Magnetotherapy. I. Title.
  R733 .L955 2003
  615.5—dc21
                                            2003057612

Table of Contents

Acknowledgments

In the field of manufacturing when a product has been started, it is called a "work in process." Unlimited Energy has been a "work in process" for over seven years. During this time many people helped in writing this book. A story that I heard once about geese comes to mind when I think of my team. I would like to share it with you.

Lessons from Geese

In the fall of the year, you will hear a commotion coming from the sky. You will look up and see them—Geese—flying in a "V" formation. You always know they are geese by their "V" pattern in the sky. Old Timers look up at them and talk about the kind of winter we are going to have. A sort of haunting feeling comes across you as you consider what was said.

Geese are incredibly intelligent creatures. This "V" formation just happens to be the most efficient way for a group to fly. Do you suppose they figured it out by themselves? I choose to think God gave them the knowledge.

As each bird flaps its wings, it creates uplift for the bird following. Flying in a "V" formation, the entire flock adds 71 percent greater flying range than if the bird flew alone.

This action reminds me of my team getting more accomplished together than could otherwise be accomplished alone. People sharing a common direction and sense of community get where they are going quicker and easier because they are traveling on the thrust of one another. Over the course of the more than seven years, team members left, died, or lost interest.

My mother was the greatest loss. Based on their position on my team, I felt emptiness as I strove to somehow go on without them. I lost friends and family members who no longer seemed to have time for me. Some came back into the formation on my team. Some didn't.

When a goose falls out of formation, it feels the drag and resistance of trying to fly alone and quickly gets back into formation to take advantage of the lifting power of the bird immediately in front.

If we have as much sense as a goose, we will stay in formations with those who are headed where we want to go and will be willing to accept their help, as well as give ours to others.

When the lead goose gets tired, it rotates back into formation and another goose flies at the point position. It pays to take turns doing the hard tasks and sharing the leadership.

My team has been a constant source of encouragement. They got me going when I didn't feel like it. They challenged me. They reminded me what would happen if I quit.

The geese in formations honk from behind to encourage those up front to keep up their speed. We need to make sure our honking from behind is encouraging and not destructive. When a goose gets sick or wounded or is shot down, two geese drop out of formation and follow it down to help and protect it. They stay with it until it is able to fly again or dies.

Then they launch out on their own with another formation, or they catch up with the flock. If we have as much sense as geese, we, too, will stand by each other in difficult times as well as when we are strong.

—these references were taken from the writings of Milton Olsen

Now I would like you to meet my team

My greatest source of inspiration, my biggest cheerleader, and my partner is my husband, *Lew*. His love, respect, and admiration for me have been unstoppable for over 36 years. I have an entrepreneurial mind sometimes filled with crazy, hare-brained ideas. Regardless, Lew takes me seriously and allows the creativity to flow. I can't imagine getting anything accomplished without him.

I have two wonderful children whom I love dearly and equally. I will mention my first-born first—*Jack*. He followed his father's example in the way he trusts and believes in me. He added to my ideas and dreams, and together we made some of them happen. Jack is everything a son should be. Living his life honorably—even in his teen-age years—he has no need for apologies or shame. He is my best friend, and I'm happy he has become my business partner.

This book would not have been completed without my daughter, *Loni*. She joined the team working on this book as editor. You are reading this book because of her. She is the team member with both feet on the ground.

Loni is the kind of person who is vital to any team. I love this little girl—this lady—with all my heart. I am so proud of the way she conducts herself in business and life with great poise and confidence. I appreciate her invaluable contribution.

Carrie Brettingen, one of our company managers, took over the operation of our marketing manufacturing company. This allowed me to focus solely on this book. It is a wonderful thing to have someone you can put your trust in. Her contribution is greatly appreciated.

Jessica Cherry played a tremendous role in helping to produce this book. She made decisions as to which alternative therapy we should include and which we should omit. She was always dependable in the large task of proof reading, even to the point of taking the work home. Thank you Jessica for doing such a good job.

Others who inspired me are *Dr. Paul Zane Pilzer*, author of *Unlimited Wealth,* who played on our team without knowing it. This book was a great source of inspiration that actually gave me a reason to write *Unlimited Energy.*

I had been in economics classes learning Keynes Economics and was getting depressed hearing about scarce resources and how hopeless things are. I was convinced the world had little, if any hope. Dr. Pilzer pointed out that through technology there are virtually unlimited resources and, therefore, unlimited wealth.

Anthony Robbins has been my mentor and coach for ten years as well as a source of encouragement and strength. He showed me how to get myself in the state I needed to be in to write this book and to take action.

Anthony showed me that it was all right to push myself and demand more from myself than any other person would ever expect. This book would not have been written without him. I appreciate his contribution.

The people who have sent me information to expand my body of research and knowledge are numerous

A mere mention of your name does not fully honor your contribution or do it justice.

Ray and Pam McCutcheon

Rodney Jones

Dr. Sam Post

Pat Bartel

Sue Robinson

Pauline J. Plourd

Jane K.

Ronnie Patton

Rod Summitt

Roy Bryant

Anne

Anne Lafferty

Tom Reynolds

Raymond Carlage

Bill

Francis Mumma

Gary Richmond

Annie Grooms

Carl Frech

James Lehman

Dr. Rodney Hard

Charles Brumbaugh

Becky Brumbaugh

Pam Hilton

Ruth Belk

Lynn Crawford

Irene Kulchytsky

Jerry Ulrich

Rick Roocroft

Elmer Hansen

I apologize to anyone whose name I have missed.

Chapter One

Choose Your Health Strategy

Never before in the history of the world have we had so many choices. We have volumes of well-written information. Anyone who can read can become his or her own doctor with great success. Of this vast number of choices, I, with the help of my assistant, have selected a few from the book entitled *Alternative Medicine* written by the Burton Group. We have read the section on the specific therapy, and restated it in our own words in an effort to make it clearer. But before we start, let us first take a look at the big picture. Let's define our objective. We do not want someone to stick needles in us merely for the sake of sticking needles in us. We do not just want to eat bitter things or swallow handfuls of capsules. We do not want to merely go through the motions of different therapies. We have an idea of what we want to accomplish when using alternative strategies--getting better, and feeling better and stronger. If the strategy is working, how do we know?

Working out a reasonable strategy for our health is similar to a general who creates a plan of attack. Generals don't commit all their troops to one battle all at once. They develop a plan that hopefully leads to a great victory. The victory must be clearly defined, or troops will founder under in confusion. A victory could be obtained, and if everyone is in the midst of confusion, no one will notice. Or, if a victory is not obtained, perhaps the plan wasn't followed up on as it should have been.

The same is true with your health. You need to develop a plan and then follow through with it. Even when your doctor gives you a prescription, you buy it, determine how to take it, and you take the medicine. However, if you are going to be your own doctor, you must, as well, devise a plan and follow through with that plan. If you don't follow through with your plan, you can't blame the "strategy" when things aren't working.

In a battle, the general calculates the risk. The greater the general, the more he or she will suffer when committing men's and women's lives into battle. The greater the general, the greater the ability to find the strategy with the lowest risk factor that will provide the best results.

Likewise, as you consider alternative strategies, be sure to make your decision with your eyes open. Consider the risks and cost, not only in money but also in time and effort. And consider any bodily discomfort that may be incurred. Select the strategy with the lowest risk for the greatest reward.

Of course, your goal is to get better, but getting better means different things to different people. You need to first define what you mean by "getting better." Then keep records, just like your doctor does. Be professional. One way of keeping score of how you are getting better is to quantify your condition. On a scale of one to ten, what is your level of pain? Do this for each area of your body. Write down your answers.

Next, evaluate the level of pain. Is it different than when you started noticing it? How? Is the pain greater? Is the pain less? Some strategies for some conditions cause initial pain at first. If you are trying the strategy for the first time, you must consider this aspect before your eliminate the strategy. Every one of these alternative medicine strategies has the same goal—to heal. However, healing is never accomplished unless energy is present. Energy is a vague term that is really not specific. Energy is movement of circling force fields. Force fields are basically the same for all energy, with a few exceptions which may vary.

- direction of the spin
- speed of the spin
- distance it travels
- size of the circle it makes in the spin

Healing energy is the same regardless of the alternative medicine strategy. At the site of all healing is a force field spinning counterclockwise, within a certain frequency and power range, and with a uni-direction (uni-pole) energy pattern. The goal of each strategy is to heal. Healing does not occur unless healing energy is present, which the body naturally manufactures.

Sometimes the body is weakened for a variety of reasons. Thus, it cannot adequately heal and may need outside assistance. This outside assistance must generate healing energy for it to work. If properly designed, therapeutic magnets bypass all these alternative medicine strategies and place this healing energy right at the site where it is needed. With magnetic therapy, your chances of success are greater than with any other strategy, with virtually no risk. Magnetic therapy, then, should be your first choice.

To better understand this process, let's take a look at something in everyday life we can see and understand. Then we will make a comparison to the body and healing.

First, let's consider a water pipe with water flowing through it. When the water stops, there are only two, possibly three, reasons.

First, there could be a problem with the water. It may be filled with mud or frozen. Our goal, then, is to get the water flowing again. If we think the problem is mud, we would place a filter on the incoming supply. If we think the problem is that the water is frozen, then we must apply heat to the pipe.

Secondly, there could be a problem with the pipe. The pipe itself may be worn and deteriorated. It may also have bent inward, which could block the flow of water. There may, as well, be holes causing the water to leak out. The inside surfaces may be jagged so particles in the water stick to the inside of the pipe. Forces outside the pipe may be exerting enough pressure to collapse the pipe.

To solve these problems, first view the system as a whole. Consider how the system works and make a list of the possible causes based on your knowledge of the system. Then make a list of things to try. Start with the simple things first. If they don't work, go to the harder things. Remember to create your plan as you go along. Ask questions: What are you going to try? How long are you going to try something before you decide it is not working? How do you know if it is or is not working?

There could be another reason the water is not flowing through the pipe. Perhaps someone shut the water off. While the solution may sound simple--just turn the water back on-- it may not be that simple. There could be hundreds of places to turn off the water. What does a water pipe have to do with the body? Plenty. Remember that there are only three possible reasons that cause circulation to be stopped or slowed.

1) There is a problem with the fluid.

The body has many filters called organs to strain out foreign particles. Some examples are the liver and tonsils. These filters are organs made of muscles. If a muscle is exercised, it becomes bigger. If these filters are too small to do their job, they get bigger. But with these filtering organs, there is a limit to how large they can become and still fit in their proper place in the body. When they reach beyond their intended size limit, they start to malfunction. The poisons and other foreign particles and other microorganisms build up pressure and slow down. This process damages the system.

Scavengers come to the rescue and consume this poison so the organ can function. To assist them, the body's pH in that area turns acidic. If this fails and the filtering organs are still not functioning properly, the body uses other emergency systems. These emergency systems are only intended to work short term because they were not designed to replace the other organs. If these emergency measures fail, the body is in trouble. This trouble is called sickness or disease.

Treating this organ with magnetic therapy could immediately start to restore circulation. As circulation improves, the poison will disappear. The scavengers will no longer be needed, and they will die due to lack of food and the elevated pH. Little by little the organ will begin to function properly. The other emergency systems will stop and let the organ take over completely. To solve this problem with the fluid, you must condition it. One way is through prescription drugs. Another is with food-- vitamins or minerals. And, the last way is with exercise.

2) There is a problem with the pipe.

Pipes are the mechanism which carry water. In the body, the pipes carry fluids. They are the body's circulatory systems. If they aren't working properly, something has restricted this process. The circulatory system can include: the blood vessels, the nerves carrying electrical signals, the lymphatic system, and the urinary tract. Here again we have only so many possible causes. To develop a strategy that can solve the problem, we first need to make a list and examine each item for possible causes. Eventually we will find the one causing the problem. In my opinion, the first place to start is to look at the posture of the body, which could be crimping shut these bodily pipes.

Stand in front of a mirror. Shoulders and hips should be parallel to the ground. There should be a straight line from the top of the head to the feet, with the shoulders in that line. If they are not, investigate ways to align and balance them.

Magnetic therapy has been known to solve alignment problems. Alignment problems can create areas of pain in the body. To solve this problem, place a properly designed therapeutic magnet directly over any painful spot so the energy from the magnet can work with the body and assist the body in restoring weak or damaged muscle. Once the muscle is strong enough and can support a weak area, pressure is removed from the bodily pipe and circulation is restored. Try it. There are no harmful side effects. Just remember to identify the real problem. The real problem must be solved before real results occur.

3) The supply could have been shut off.

For this book, we are using the term strategy to mean a plan of action. You are devising a plan of action that you will follow through with to solve a health problem. There are long-term strategies that lay out the action for years and years at a time. There are also short-term strategies that lay out the action for a few days or weeks or a couple of months.

Magnetic therapy falls into the long-term strategy category. Magnets can assist the body in healing itself, and they can also keep a healthy body healthy. Magnets provide people with extra energy. In fact, we humans get 30 percent of our energy from sources (magnetic energy) other than through food. Of course, good diet and exercise are other examples of long term strategies.

Magnetic therapy is also a short-term strategy. Sometimes one can place the magnet directly over a recent injury and the pain goes away in seconds. Even in traditional therapies, short-term strategies are not intended to be used long-term. Surgery is a short-term strategy. So is drug therapy. One should not go through one surgery after another in an ongoing fashion. Surgery is designed to solve a problem. Nor should one live a life dependent on drugs. And, keep in mind that many traditional therapies can work well with magnetic therapy. Some can help magnetic therapy work more efficiently.

Magnetic therapy is particularly useful when working with structural problems. A person's bone structure must be balanced and strong if it is to support the body. God designed our bodies so the strong muscles of the body are in place to do this work. When these muscles weaken, our bodily structure is not properly supported. Nerves become pinched. You can place magnets directly over the pain, and it can help. But the real solution is not to increase circulation at the site of the pain but to increase circulation at the source of the problem.

Remember that if you have an obstructed water line, you have two ways to repair it. You can increase the pressure to move the blockage, or you can make the water line larger. Either one will increase circulation. Likewise, the term "alternative medicine" provides more than one solution. There are different strategies for getting healthy and staying healthy. The very term "alternative" holds an underlying assumption. This assumption suggest that there exist a solid body of strategies--strategies that are alternative to traditional strategies. There are those used by the established medical community, such as surgery and drug therapy. Then there are more, untested, under-researched alternatives. It is also assumed that established medical practices are not only "choices" but are also accepted as the foundation of our medical culture and are often not questioned. Because the methods are not questioned, they are no longer scientific. Unquestioned medical strategies have turned into marketing. Marketers of traditional therapies protect their territory and take advantage of the great respect they have become accustomed to, and they continually attempt to further elevate their status.

For purposes of this publication, we will accept this assumption and continue to call the so-called, untested, under-researched health strategies "alternative medicine," but we do so only for communication. We do not believe these methods are merely alternatives. We believe they stand shoulder to shoulder with surgery and drug therapy and all the other methods used in established medicine.

Why? Because these so-called "alternatives" are not untested nor are they unresearched. In fact, some of these methods have more research and testing then some mainstream medical strategies. Some so-called "alternative" strategies have withstood the test of time because they have been in use for thousands of years. Millions of people are benefiting from them.

So, when considering a specific therapy, consider a number of things. First of all, consider the risk. What if you make a mistake? How can misapplying the therapy hurt you? Is the risk worth it? Other things to consider are the effectiveness, the cost, how hard it is to learn, and how it fits into your life-style. Magnetic therapy may end up being the number one choice of all therapies when viewed this way. There is no risk if the magnet is a properly designed therapeutic magnet and if it is used correctly. It cannot hurt you. If magnetic therapy fails, there can be only four reasons.

- incorrect pole or energy pattern
- magnets are not strong enough

- magnets are not used long enough
- magnets are placed in the wrong location

Magnets can be 100-percent effective. They are also very inexpensive because properly designed therapeutic magnets last at least 30 years. The technology is easy to learn. Getting started is as easy as placing the magnet directly over the painful area. There are products available to fit any lifestyle.

The following "alternatives" are presented in an unusual order. They are listed according to how they work. My reasoning focuses on the body's circulation; therefore, I have arranged the therapies according to the role they play in restoring circulation. Some therapies work on all three problems. They can condition fluid that is delivered, they can repair the passageway, or they can turn on the system, while predominantly focusing on one problem. Other therapies may focus on only one. They either condition fluid to be delivered, repair the passageway, or turn the system on.

If magnetic fields are not used, nothing happens. Problems persist and worsen. The goal of all therapies is to create these force fields. So, it's a matter of choosing which one you want to use to obtain and maintain good health.

Conditioning the Fluid

Chemical Change

Diet

Doctors agree that diet plays an important role in a person's overall health, but achieving a good diet is not easy. Just because we eat what we believe to be the right foods doesn't guarantee that we are obtaining the right kind or the right amount of nutrition. The problem is that we simply don't know what harmful contaminants are present in foods we eat. Seldom do we know where the food is grown or raised and what chemicals are present in it. Thus, our bodies, simply by our eating a variety of foods grown on a number of soils, receive contaminants and chemicals that may pose health risks.

Benefits

A good diet of whole foods promotes health by decreasing fat and sugar while increasing fiber and nutrients. Such a diet means we will eat less, which reduces the chances of gaining excess weight. The key to better health is to eat more fiber. Fiber is the transport system of the digestive tract, moving food wastes from the body before it has a chance to form potentially cancer-causing and mutagenic chemicals. These toxic chemicals may cause colon cancer or pass through the gastrointestinal membrane into the bloodstream and damage other cells.

Author's Opinion

Eating a whole-foods diet is not merely a health strategy but is a way of life. It just makes common sense to nourish the body. At a gas station, you pay more for high-energy fuel for your car, so why would you fill your body with low-energy fuel when you can get high-energy fuel for the same price? My personal principle regarding food is simple. I eat what I need for the work or activity I am about to do. I notice that if I eat a so-called normal breakfast of eggs, toast, and beef sausage, I become lethargic. To avoid this problem, I eat a small amount of high-energy food such as tofu, scrambled like eggs, along with some kind of vegetable such as broccoli. This nontraditional breakfast is loaded with nutrients. It gives me instant energy that sustains me all morning. It nourishes my mind for clear thinking. I feel great.

Listen to your body. What do you like? Why are you eating? Eat what you need to enable you to perform at your peak for the hours that will follow a meal. Keep records to remember which foods provided the necessary energy needed to complete a task.

Nutritional Supplements

If you are like me, you will not depend on or trust your eating choices—excellent though they may be—to supply all the nutrients necessary for excellent health. Even traditional medical persons are beginning to agree that nutritional supplements are necessary to cure a variety of illnesses, injuries, and age-related problems. I have even heard medical experts say that vitamin and mineral supplements help to maintain optimal physical and psychological health and promote longevity and chronic disease prevention.

It has been said and it is true: we are digging our graves with our teeth. This is due to over-consumptive undernutrition. In other words, we are eating empty-calorie foods. We may eat enough of the right foods, but two-thirds of an average American's diet is made up of fats and refined sugars. As a result, the average American is nutrient deficient. This can help destroy the body's natural resistance to disease and premature aging while also weakening physiological and psychological performance.

Benefits

Not getting the proper nutrition can lead to such problems as lassitude, fatigue, mood swings, insomnia, and many other conditions with no clear diagnosis. Vitamins are also critical in the treatment of cataracts, heart disease, high blood pressure, and cancer.

Author's Opinion

The recent technological advancements in food supplements are incredible. Modern food supplements are more easily absorbed by the body, are inexpensive, and are easy to take. For the best health choices possible, investigate and study the product lines of several suppliers. Apply common sense and use what makes sense to you. After about a week of taking a new supplement, decide whether or not it is working. You should notice some kind of benefit. If not, ask questions. You may conclude that this particular formula is not right for you. If that is the case, then you should discontinue use and find another supplement. Apply the same principle as one uses when investing on Wall Street: Ditch the losers—Run with the winners. It is just that simple.

Juice Therapy

Yes, there are some medical doctors that actually treat certain illnesses and diseases with nothing but juice. This treatment is based on the ability of the raw juice of vegetables and fruits to nourish and replenish the body. In certain prescriptions, vegetable, fruit, and herb juice are used during periods of stress and illness. In addition, juice therapy is also used as part of a comprehensive health maintenance plan because it is an excellent way to supplement the diet. Drinking juice can also aid patients in other treatment programs because juice therapy stimulates the immune system. For example, it can help treat blood pressure problems and can detoxify the body. Juice is also successful in the treatment of food allergies and is great for people with nausea or digestive problems. In some applications of juice therapy, a system of cleansing and restoration follows, and the fresh juices provide a nutritional foundation to help the body heal itself. Generally, fresh juices are quite versatile in any curative or maintenance program.

Benefits

Many doctors use juice therapy in conjunction with fasts and as nutritional supplementation for diseases such as allergies and arthritis or as part of a treatment of cancer and AIDS. Juices of fresh fruits and vegetables contain a rich supply of enzymes. When fruits and vegetables are juiced, their enzymes are released and immediately go to work when they are consumed. This aids the body in its constant work of dissolving and eliminating wastes as well as speeding delivery of the vital nutrients contained in the juices.

Homeopathy

No alternative presentation of health strategies would be complete without homeopathy. Homeopathy is no different from all the other strategies in that its goal is to get healing energy to the site where it is needed.

The following excerpt is taken from *Discovery of Magnetic Health* by George J. Washnis: "Many believe that homeopathic remedies are essentially pure electromagnetic energies, derived from various crude substances used to jump-start the healing process. They function as any counterirritant would, such as a mustard plaster, for example. After a number of steps, the form, smell, and color of the original substances are lost in the final product.

"In the end, products cannot be differentiated from one another. The final substance, which replicates ingredients of the original ailment, is so diluted that it heals rather than creates symptoms, by either manufacturing a negative magnetic field or attracting negative energy to that locale. All drugs are removed; only the memory of the energy remains.

Even the founder of homeopathy, Samuel Hahnermann, recognized magnetic energy as a principle of homeopathic effectiveness. What is extremely fascinating about homeopathy and magnetotherapy is that they both rely to a large extent on magnetic energy. Millions of people use the healing power of homeopathy, never realizing that it very likely employs the principle of attracting negative magnetic energy to the injury.

"Medical doctors and many other specialists have never understood how a homeopath could take a substance and dilute it to such an extent that there is no measurement of ingredients left, yet healing or relief takes place.

Dr. William Philpott, who has helped thousands of individuals using homeopathic methods for a period of years, believes that what is taking place is a reversal of the magnetic field in the substance from a positive polarity to a negative polarity or the attraction of the negative field to the area by the homeopathic substance. In fact, Philpott says that he has stopped using the rather complex assortment of homeopathic substances designed for specific diseases and ailments. He simply applies magnetotherapy with equally effective results, since these therapies are designed to achieve the same effect but by different procedures.

"If the similarity between homeopathy and magnetotherapy holds true, this would be a most fascinating discovery, making magnetotherapy all the more relevant for its comparative simplicity and higher degree of predictability. It does not mean that the homeopath should discard this procedure for the more simple magnetotherapy, since each type of therapy has its own intrinsic values. Homeopathy has physical and mental attributes and feelings or beliefs that can be beneficial to particular patients. It does mean, however, that magnetotherapy could very well fit into the regimen of homeopathy and possibly make treatment successful in a higher percentage of cases by a clearer understanding of how it can be applied to achieve specific result[s], by varying strength and exposure time.

Homeopathy may work more quickly in certain circumstances depending on the substance and the extent of dilution. The two methodologies can work hand-in-hand.

Most importantly, this observation and understanding can help reduce the skepticism of physicians in order to allow them to consider the use of these therapies.

"In short, homeopathy is a function of succession and dilution, where the succession or jarring of solution can create static negative electricity of positive magnetic energy poled that perform very much like any other irritant to stimulate the functioning of the counterirritant immune system. Each homeopathic remedy carries a very weak magnetic field that relieves a particular symptom by attracting negative ions to the site and allowing the immune system to build resistance to the substance so that the body can better tolerate it. Various levels of dilution give the body time to react with the least stress possible."

Herbal Medicine

"Here, eat this root." "No, eat this plant."

These are two familiar pieces of advice from medicine men of the past. Herbal medicine is the most ancient form of health care, but modern science is just now beginning to see its benefits and is now studying herbal treatments for nearly every disease. Herbal medicine works similar to conventional pharmaceutical drugs.

However, herbs contain large numbers of naturally occurring chemicals that have biological activity. Because herbs and plants use an indirect route to the bloodstream and target organs, their effects are usually slower and less dramatic than drugs.

Herbal medicine works best when used to facilitate healing in chronic ongoing problems. By skillfully selecting herbs, a profound transformation in health can be effected with less danger of the side effects inherent in drug-based medicine.

Benefits

Herbal remedies can be used for a wide range of minor ailments that are amenable to self-medication: stomach upset, the common cold, the flu, minor aches and pains, constipation and diarrhea, coughs, headaches, menstrual cramps, digestive disturbances, sore muscles, skin rashes, sunburn, dandruff, and insomnia. Other conditions that respond well to herbal medicine include digestive disorders, such as peptic ulcers, colitis, and irritable bowel syndrome; rheumatic and arthritic conditions; chronic skin problems, such as eczema and psoriasis; problems of the menstrual cycle and especially premenstrual syndrome; anxiety and tension-related stress; bronchitis and other respiratory conditions; hypertension; and allergies. According to Dr. Alex Guerrero, herbal medicines can be used as treatment for any disease or disorder.

Author's Opinion

The Bible speaks of using bitter herbs for medicine, and this health strategy is worth considering. The upside is that this treatment is natural, effective, and inexpensive.

The down side is that it is somewhat complicated, some herbs may be hard to find, and there is a risk if they are not used properly.

Fasting

When fasting, one eats nothing and drinks a good deal of water. Fasting is a tried-and-true and effective therapy for a wide range of conditions, including hypertension, headaches, allergies, and arthritis. By relieving the body of the task of digesting foods, fasting allows the system to rid itself of toxins while facilitating healing. A great deal of energy is needed to break food down into its nutritional components, convert food's carbohydrates and proteins into glycogen (a starch which can be converted into energy) for storage in the liver, and provide the body with the fuel necessary to perform its functions.

When the intake of calories is restricted or eliminated, the body fuels itself through alternate means. During the first two days of a fast, the liver converts stored sugars into glucose that the body can use for fuel. When these stores are depleted, fat is used as a source of energy. Fasting aids most health concerns because during a fast, without the extra work of digesting food, the body is free to get rid of stored toxins. Since new toxins are not coming in with food, the body can concentrate on cleansing itself very efficiently. The immune system works better and can handle allergic reactions and inflammations more effectively.

By the fourth day, the blood thins and increases oxygen to tissues which brings more white blood cells to the body. Because energy is freed to do other things, the self-regulation systems function better. These include the immune, growth, and elimination systems. Stored fat becomes the primary source of energy. As this fat moves out, so do chemicals from pesticides and drugs—straight to the now more efficient elimination system.

The body has the natural ability to recognize old, nonessential tissues and dissolve them. Any usable nutrients in the tissue are employed for new cell production.

With more elimination, more efficient physiological function results. Fasting creates a different, more aware, more sensitive focus of gratitude for one's surroundings. It is a spiritual experience as well as an enhancement to health.

Benefits

Heart disease, hypertension, arthritis, allergies, inflammatory diseases, psychological problems, and headache problems can be helped when one fasts. Allergies, respiratory diseases, and acute illnesses are most responsive to a fast, while chronic degenerative diseases are less responsive, often requiring several repeated fasts.

Author's Opinion

Isaiah 5:8 says that if people fast, their health will spring back speedily. This is an excellent example of fasting's benefit. Fasting gives the body a rest and, therefore, gives it the ability to heal itself.

Hydrotherapy

Hydrotherapy is the use of water, ice, steam, and hot and cold temperatures to maintain and restore health. Treatments include full-body immersion, steam baths, saunas, sitz baths, colonic irrigation, and the application of hot and/or cold compresses. It is used for a wide range of conditions and can be administered at home.

Benefits

Hydrotherapy has been used to treat disease and injury by many different cultures for many centuries. It is very effective in ridding the body of poisons and toxins. External hydrotherapies fall into three categories: hot water, cold water, or contrast. Each gives a specific result. Heat relaxes and creates a response in the body that stimulates the immune system. It causes white blood cells to travel from the blood stream and into tissues so they can eliminate toxins. Hot water also soothes and relaxes, benefiting every organ and system of the body.

Cold water stimulates. It reduces inflammation by constricting the blood vessels. Inflammatory agents are reduced, thus making the blood vessels less permeable. And cold water tones muscles. For a fever, cold water drives the fever slightly up at first but lowers it in the long term.

Oxygen Therapy

For the body to turn food into energy, oxygen must be present, and many health problems are often something as simple as a lack of oxygen. To list oxygen's benefits would be a difficult task. Virtually every illness and disease would need to be included. As a brief explanation, we can say that oxygen therapy promotes healing and assists the body in healing itself. Therapies are grouped according to the chemical process involved. The addition of oxygen to blood or tissues is called oxygenation. An example is hyperbaric oxygen therapy which involves the use of a pressurized chamber.

Oxidation is the reaction of splitting off electrons from any chemical molecule. Oxidation sometimes involves oxygen and sometimes it doesn't. It is a chemical reaction. Hydrogen peroxide therapy is an example of the use of the process of oxidation.

If cells do not have enough oxygen, parasites can thrive and reproduce. If the body has too much oxygen through the hyperbaric high-pressure process, tissues could be damaged. Oxygenation administered correctly by knowledgeable people results in saturating the body with oxygen and is very beneficial.

Benefits

Oxygen therapy is primarily used for traumas, such as crash injuries, burns, wounds, gangrene (death of tissue, usually due to deficient or absent blood supply), carbon monoxide poisoning, bed sores, stasis (the stagnation of the normal flow of fluids), radiation necrosis (death of an area of tissue or bone surrounded by healthy parts), and recalcitrant skin grafting (skin grafting that doesn't take). Some microsurgical procedures for the repair and restoration of severed limbs are made possible only by the use of oxygen therapy during the surgery.

Chelation Therapy

Chelation therapy is administered by injecting a chelating agent into the blood stream. This substance removes calcium plaque from the artery walls, increasing blood flow. It also gets rid of toxic and metabolic metals as well as unnecessary metals. As a result, hardening of the arteries or atherosclerosis is reversed. This therapy is safe and effective in preventing heart attacks and strokes and is an alternative to bypass surgery and angioplasty. When circulation is restored, many conditions are helped.

Chelation therapy has been successful in reversing gangrene, alleviating leg cramps, and restoring memory. Because it removes toxic metal ions, it reduces internal inflammation caused by free radicals. It can ease symptoms of degenerative diseases including arthritis, lupus, and scleroderma.

Chelation therapy is performed on an outpatient basis, is painless, and takes approximately three and a half hours. For optimal results, physicians who use chelation therapy recommend twenty to thirty treatments given at an average rate of one to three per week, with patient evaluations being made at regular intervals. The patient reclines comfortably and is given an intravenous solution of EDTA with vitamins and minerals.

Benefits

One study documented significant improvement in 99% of patients suffering from peripheral vascular disease and blocked arteries of the legs. Twenty-four percent of those patients with cerebrovascular and other degenerative cerebral diseases also showed marked improvement, with an additional 30% having good improvement. Overall, nearly 90% of all treated patients have marked or good improvement with chelation therapy.

Author's Opinion

The goal of this therapy is to restore circulation, but in my opinion, this is an unnatural process. There are many better and healthier methods of improving the circulation of fluids in the body. Another negative is that a specialist is required to administer the treatment. What is the main focus here? Is it needed treatment or a steady cash flow for the therapist? I am not attempting to condemn or make assumptions, but keep in mind that the main goal of chelation therapy is to restore circulation. To restore circulation, I feel that magnetic therapy is a better choice.

Colon Therapy

Colon therapy rids the intestinal track of caked-in fecal matter that may have been stuck in folds of the inner walls of the intestines for several years. As a result, the body's chemistry is brought into balance, and this restores the proper function of the colon.

Author's Opinion

The goal of this therapy is to restore proper circulation. This therapy works like a high-pressure hose flushing out clogged mud. If the person has a huge build-up of waste material that will not pass naturally, then this would be the best way to eliminate it. But I know of cases where properly designed therapeutic magnets placed over the colon for a specified period of time produced the same results.

Repairing the Passageway

Energy Medicine

Energy medicine really isn't a therapy but several diagnostic screening devices. These devices measure the energy being emitted from the body in specific areas. The goal is to detect irregularities of the energy, whether an imbalance or a blockage. The theory is that if energy is returned to what is thought to be normal, a healthy state will result.

Once a specific area is pin-pointed, other therapies are then used to treat the body. These diagnostic systems are electrocardiogram, electroencephalogram, eletromyelogram and MRI (magnetic resonance imaging). Their greatest goal is to detect problems early enough to successfully treat them. The closely-related field of bioenergy therapy is the actual treatment of disease. Examples of these therapies are electrical, magnetic, sonic, acoustic, microware and infrared.

Energy Medicine Devices

These bioenergy therapy systems use an acupuncture meridian system. A meridian is nothing more than a passageway or a highway for energy to travel. This is not just a helter-skelter series of passageways but is a charitable system that is the same in every body. When the energy doesn't flow freely through the meridians, organs or other parts of the body depending on that energy become stressed and break down. Thus illness or disease can begin to take hold. As a road map shows how different highways go to different cities, different organs are supplied with energy by different meridians. Acupuncture points are like junctions in highways. They are also like control points along a highway, and energy at the acupoints can be measured and manipulated. Thus, they are known as control measurement points.

Treatment Instruments

Once the diagnosis is made with the electroacupuncture biofeedback devices, the treatment can begin. The goal is to restore or balance the flow of energy. A list of these devices includes the Mora, the TENS Unit, the Electro-Acuscope, the Light Beam Generator (LBG), the Sound Probe, the Diapulse,

Cymatic Instruments, the Infratonic QGM, and the Teslar Watch.

Author's Opinion

What is an energy imbalance? The only characteristic of energy that can be out of balance is the amount of north pole energy and south pole energy. An energy imbalance is almost always excessive south pole energy. Let's take an example of an injury. South pole energy floods the area. As it spreads, so does pain. This is why the whole area hurts when an injury occurs in one spot. The body responds by directing north pole energies to the site. Sometimes it must take energy away from the body's normal functions, and, as a result, the person may feel faint. As soon as the body restores a balance of north and south pole energy, the pain goes away. Work is underway to replace the damaged cells with new healthy ones, and when this work is completed, the injury is healed.

The easiest, fastest, most effective way to treat energy imbalances is with magnets. If there is excessive south pole energy, you supply the site with more powerful north pole energy. How simple can it get? These diagnostic devices all work basically the same. They scan the body or area and in one way or another, read the excessive south pole energies and communicate the readings to the specialist, showing the areas of imbalance. The cause could be anything from cancer to an infection. The specialist or therapist then asks the patient questions and suggests a probable cause for the imbalance.

The goal of all aspects of this therapy is the same: to deliver healing energy to the site where it is needed by cleaning out congested electrical highways.

However, for a responsible person setting out to be his or her own doctor, most methods are impractical. The machines or equipment are too expensive and difficult to find. Even if they were affordable and easy to find, they are difficult to learn to use. The user also runs the risk of administering the treatment incorrectly, which could result in injury. While this area of health strategy is fascinating and experts are using these methods with success, there are better and more effective choices. Magnetic therapy is a better choice. Everything that is accomplished with these cumbersome methods is just as effectively accomplished with magnetic therapy without the cost, risk, or the complicated instructions. The only negative to magnetic therapy is there are no quantitative results. In other words, you can't see the test numbers improve as you can with one of the above measuring devices.

Chiropractic

Chiropractic treatment became part of mainstream medicine with the treatment of whiplash. The most traditional method for treating whiplash was traction, which lasted several painful days. Other treatments that adjusted the spine and joints had some success. As chiropractic treatments gained recognition, more and more were routinely performed for a large number of ailments. Successful treatment of back problems, headaches, injuries, traumas, and many disorders have made chiropractic treatment the second largest primary health care field in the world.

The focus of chiropractic treatment is on the relationship of the spinal column and the musculoskeletal structures of the body to the nervous system, which holds the key to the body's incredible potential to heal itself because it coordinates and controls the functions of all the other systems. The theory behind the science of chiropractic treatment is that the proper alignment of the spinal column is essential for optimum health because it acts as a "switchboard" for the nervous system.

When there is interference caused by misalignment in the spine, known as subluxation, pain can occur and the body's defenses can be diminished. By adjusting the spinal joints to remove subluxation, normal nerve function can be restored. The spine as a whole operates as a functional unit; each vertebra can affect its neighbor, and one portion of the spine may affect or damage other areas of the body. Subluxation of the spinal vertebrae can also affect the body in less obvious ways. A subluxation can have a direct effect on an organ's function when it impedes the proper nerve flow to that organ. When the vertebrae are properly aligned, the spine remains mobile, allowing electrical impulses from the brain to travel freely along the spinal cord to the organs, thus maintaining healthy function. However, when subluxation occurs, it interrupts the normal flow in the nerve structures and that, in turn, affects the normal functioning of the organ.

Benefits

These treatments can help maintain the overall heath of the nervous system and the organs. Treatments started directly after serious injury can decrease the accumulation of scar formation, which can prevent later weakening or stiffness of any joints affected.

Author's Opinion

The goal of this therapy is to restore proper circulation of the body's electrical highways. When circulation is restricted, the body is in pain. Through manipulation, the chiropractor relieves pain or pressure, and a skillful chiropractor can do this quickly. The drawback is that often the original condition returns, and patients must repeat treatments.

Acupuncture

With a 1970s study, researchers concluded that acupuncture

points boosted the electrical signals traveling through the body. They thought that the insertion of a needle interfered with energy flow and blocked the stimulus of pain. To most people, as well as medical practitioners, acupuncture is a complex, integrated healing system. While many admit they do not understand how acupuncture works, they have seen evidence of actual healing of a variety of conditions, including diseases of the eyes, nerves, muscle, heart as well as the digestion and reproduction organs.

Author's Opinion

I disagree with the conclusions of the 1970 study because I believe that energy is a friend and not an enemy. It is the free flow of energy that relieves pain--not the blockage of it. Based on my experience and beliefs, I am confident that I understand the working of acupuncture and believe it is very simple and easy for anyone to understand.

Within the body is an entire network of highways which transport energy. This energy has all the same characteristics of other force fields. Most of this energy is manufactured by the body and directed by the brain down the highway to where it is needed. In addition, some of this energy is taken into the body from an outside source, and this outside source is the earth. There are many places where these electrical highways cross. If we were looking at a map, we would call these places intersections or junctions. The term in this health strategy is called an acupuncture point.

Acupuncture points have more energy than places on any given stretch of electrical highway. When the body is injured, energy travels to the site of the injury in lightning speeds. The goal of the acupuncturist is to get the body to direct a blast of energy to this point. Acupuncturists do this by slightly injuring the body by inserting a needle. The reason they choose a certain point as opposed to a different one is skilled acupuncturists know which points to use to get the energy where it is needed.

Acupuncture is an energy-delivery method. If you were going to Chicago, you would look at a map and select the best highways to get there. In terms of acupuncture, if you have a headache, you would look at the acupuncture map and select the right highways that lead to the head. Just like following a physical highway going to Chicago, you insert the needle at the correct acupuncture point. It is needed at the place where poor circulation problems occur, sometimes referred to as a disease or symptom such as pain. The goal of acupuncture is to get healing energy to the place it is needed. It's just that simple.

The same or at least similar results are accomplished when you place a properly designed therapeutic magnet over an acupuncture point. Properly designed means properly designed for that particular task. To gain the most from magnetic therapy, the right magnet must fit the need. The process is then fine tuned to obtain maximum results. A properly designed acupuncture point magnet is round and about five millimeters in diameter. This type of magnet sends out the force field in the shape of a cone with the point toward the body. This point is where a greater concentration of energy lies. This energy jumps on the electrical highway and is sent to the site of the problem. This treatment creates very little stress to the body and is very natural and gentle. With magnetic acupuncture, one can bypass the needles and, therefore, bypass the pain and stress caused by the needles.

With needles, the exact site is very important. If the acupuncturist does not contact the right place, the electrical energy will not travel on the right electrical highway and will not get to the correct site. When this happens, the procedure must be repeated, causing more pain and stress.

With magnets, the exact site is necessary but very forgiving when the correct point is missed. And needle-induced acupuncture must be performed by an expert, but acupuncture with magnets can be done by anyone who can read an electrical map of the body. Magnetic acupuncture is safer and less painful than traditional acupuncture. Both accomplish the same goal: getting a burst of healing energy to travel down an electrical highway to the site of a problem.

At present many acupuncturists know about enhancing their treatment with magnets. They will identify the acupuncture point on the patient's body and position the magnets directly over the marked point and usually secure them in place with tape for extended usage.

(See the chapter entitled "The Real World" to review my experiences with magnetic acupuncture.)

Applied Kinesiology

In my opinion, Applied Kinesiology is a very fascinating subject. A practitioner asks you to resist with a certain set of muscles. If your resistance is weak, the practitioner knows right where your problem is. This procedure is referred to as muscle testing. A problem in the body signals health imbalances. But applied kinesiology goes beyond muscle testing; it can diagnose and resolve a variety of health problems. Applied Kinesiology is a study of the activity of muscles and the relationship of muscle strength to health. Muscle dysfunction in an otherwise healthy person can be corrected by using various reflexes or by performing a manual procedure on the muscle, such as deep massage, goading pressure on the attachment points, or realignment. By this method, muscles can reset to function smoothly.

Author's Opinion

Incorporating magnets into this strategy will make it work more efficiently and, therefore, faster. In order for a weak organ or muscle to be strengthened, it must have the building blocks of oxygen and nutrients. These building blocks are delivered through the blood or come directly through the skin. Magnets assist their free flow to the weakness.

Aromatherapy

Aromatherapy uses a substance extracted from plants and herbs called essential oils. Essential oils are used to treat conditions ranging from infections and skin disorders to immune deficiencies and stress. The chemical makeup of essential oils gives them a host of desirable pharmacological properties ranging from antibacterial, antiviral, and antispasmodic ones, to uses as diuretics as well as to both widening and narrowing blood vessels. Essential oils act on the adrenals, ovaries, and the thyroid, and they can energize or pacify, detoxify and facilitate the digestive process.

They also are effective for treating infection. The usage of essentials oils soothes the nervous system by modifying response and harmonizing moods and emotions.

Aromatherapy works with aromatic molecules interacting with the top of the nasal cavity, giving off signals that are modified by various biological processes before traveling to the emotional switchboard of the brain, the limbic system.

There they create impressions associated with previous experiences and emotions. Because the limbic system is directly connected to those parts of the brain that control heart rate, blood pressure, breathing, memory, stress levels and hormone balance, the use of these oil fragrances may be one of the fastest ways to achieve physiological or psychological effects.

Inhaling the fragrance of certain essential oils can alter the neurochemistry of the brain to produce changes in mental and emotional behavior. Even aromas too subtle to be consciously detected can have significant effects on central nervous system activity. Matching the correct essential oil with the task can shorten performance time and may even cut it in half.

Benefits

For bacterial and viral infections, essential oils are powerful microbe-fighting agents without the side effects of antibiotics. They do not destroy intestinal bacteria, nor do they create kidney toxicity or anemia or lower white cell count.

For herpes simplex, a one-time application of either true rose oil or true melissa oil can lead to complete remission of herpes simplex lesions.

For shingles, a painful skin virus, Ravensera aromatica and Calophyllum inophyllum together, applied to the skin, have brought complete remissions in a week.

To regulate the body's heating and cooling system, the oils are used to regulate overprotective sebaceous glands which helps the body retain heat.

People report--and studies show--different essential oils being used to enhance the functioning of the nervous system and heighten mental abilities or relaxation. Advanced spa treatments include the use of essential oils for muscle spasms and the soothing of the skin and muscles.

Author's Opinion

How does it work? The aroma stimulates the brain to produce or direct healing energy to certain parts of the body where there is poor circulation. It works the same as every other therapy. The goal is to get healing energy to the site of need. Aromatherapy is completely safe and inexpensive, and a complicated diagnosis is not necessary. Anyone can use this for uplifting the spirit whether using it to get rid of disease or not. This wonderful, gentle therapy is icing on the cake, so to speak. Magnets can also stimulate the same organs that are stimulated by the aroma. The negative to Aromatherapy is that it is inexact, hit or miss. But what therapy isn't? Each body is different and has different, unique things happening to it. The key is to find what is effective for your body. To accomplish this, keep records. You may feel better after taking a lavender bath, but you can't predict the results. You can't stay in the tub forever, so the period of time in which to use this therapy is limited. Some keep the aromas in the air through burning incense or sprays, yet the effectiveness drastically declines after the first smelling. Should this be used together with other therapies? You are the doctor. It is your body. In my opinion, it should not be used exclusively. It is an enjoyable way to enhance the body's level of pleasure and to eliminate stress.

Biological Dentistry

This relatively new field specializes in the nontoxic restoration of materials for dental work. It focuses on the unrecognized impact dental toxins and hidden dental infections can have on overall health. It recognizes that mercury and other dental materials contribute to much of the degenerative diseases people seek help for today. There are five areas of this field.

1—Electro-Acupuncture Biofeedback

This procedure uses the acupuncture meridian system to screen for infections and dysfunctions in the body. It is simply this: each tooth is connected to an organ in the body. If there is a problem with a tooth, there may be a problem with the corresponding organ and vice versa.

2—Neural Therapy

The theory is basically the same as that of acupuncture. The body has a network of electrical highways delivering energy to all parts. As long as this energy flow is unimpeded and stays within its normal range, the body will remain healthy.

If these highways become clogged, disruptions in the normal function of cells can occur, eventually leading to chronic disorders. Injection of a local anesthetic, such as procaine, around the tooth to remove the energy blockage will often resolve the problem.

3—Oral Acupuncture

This is an injection of either saline water, weak local anesthetics, or sterile complex homeopathics into the specific acupuncture points of the oral mucous membrane.

4—Cold Laser Therapy

This is just like acupuncture only without the needles. Instead of needles, low power and light spectrums which are incapable of causing any thermal damage to the body's tissue are used. Cold laser therapy kills bacteria, aids in wound healing, reduces inflammation and helps rebalance the flow of energy in the body's meridian system.

5—Mouth Balancing

It is believed structural deformities of the skull influence the entire body. Special braces are made to be worn in the mouth to help realign the jaw and remove pain.

Author's Opinion

Proper investigation should be done to determine the real cause of the ailment. I liken this condition to a house with a cracked foundation and walls that are shifting and cracking. If only the walls are fixed, they will shift and crack again.

Likewise, with misalignment in the mouth, there could be a defective foundation, such as crooked hips or other problems. This misalignment telescopes up the body and throws the mouth out of alignment.

No matter how many times the problem in the mouth is repaired, it will return until the body's foundation is repaired.

Homeopathy

Homeopathy may be used to help alleviate pain or discomfort of dental emergencies until the problem can be fixed.

Nutrition

Nutritional supplements can be used in dealing with dental conditions, especially for the patient recovering from mercury amalgam toxicity. There have been no studies in the United States on the safety of mercury in dental work, but when it leaks from the teeth, it can cause both physical and mental problems. Numbness and tingling, paralysis, tremors, and pain are just some of the symptoms of chronic metal intoxication associated with the use of mercury dental amalgams. The most common reactions are found to be produced by the mercury amalgams used for fillings and by the various metal components that make them up, including mercury, copper, tin, zinc, and silver. Some of the symptoms caused specifically by amalgam fillings include:

—Chronic fatigue syndrome and lack of energy

—Tendency to chronic inflammatory changes (including rheumatoid arthritis, phlebitis, and fibromyalgia)

—Chronic neurological illnesses, especially when numbness is one of the leading symptoms

—Lowering of the pain threshold

—Disturbances of the immune system

Patients can be screened for sensitivity by a simple blood test known as the Clifford Materials Reactivity Testing. Everything used on the body is applied to the mouth. I have addressed these issues earlier. Once again, the main goal of all of these therapies is to deliver healing energy where it needs to be. Sometimes you can bypass the treatments by placing a magnet directly over the site and sometimes not. It's your call.

Bodywork

The term "bodywork" refers to therapies such as massage, deep-tissue manipulation, movement awareness, and energy balancing, which are employed to improve the structure and functioning of the human body. Bodywork in all its forms helps to reduce pain, soothe injured muscles, stimulate blood and lymphatic circulation, and promote deep relaxation.

Benefits

Bodywork can benefit such conditions as muscle spasm and pain, spinal curvatures, soreness related to injury, stress, headaches, whiplash, as well as TMJ and tension related respiratory disorders, including bronchial asthma or emphysema. It can also help reduce swelling, correct posture, improve body motion, and facilitate the elimination of toxins from the body. It also releases tension and promotes relaxation.

Light Therapy

The goal of light therapy is to regulate the body clock. Photobiologists point out that the light is registered by the eyes through the retina, which then transfers impulses to the hypothalamus in the brain to normalize the body-clock function.

Special light will help synchronize sleep/wake patterns with one's work and life style.

The amount of daylight exposure one receives and the changes in sunrise/sunset (which reduce the daylight hours in the fall and winter) can affect sufferers of Seasonal Affective Disorder (SAD). SAD is a specific type of major depression. The most commonly believed hypothesis follows: although the body has natural daily rhythms, they are not fully precise and rely on the intensity of sunlight to provide adjusting cues. These cues originate in the retina at the back of the eye, creating signals that pass through the optic nerve to the mid brain. These signals set in motion a number of chemical changes, which include:

—Increase in the neurotransmitter serotonin necessary for a sense of well being.

—Regulation and suppression of the hormone melatonin, which is a factor in normal sleep patterns and may influence sleep's recuperative benefits.

This major depression, seasonal or otherwise, is characterized by a series of symptoms which may include the following:

- change in appetite or weight
- sleep problems
- lack of energy
- diminishing sex drive
- body aches or pains
- memory loss
- inability to make decisions
- problems concentrating
- low self-esteem (feelings of worthlessness or guilt)

- lack of interest in or enjoyment of activities
- suicidal thoughts

How Can SAD Be Treated?

In many ways, the treatment of SAD is similar to that of other major depressive episodes, utilizing antidepressant or mood stabilizing medication and/or psychotherapy. In addition, the exposure to bright light has been found to be an effective means of treating seasonal affective disorder. The individual sits in front of a bright light unit, a specialized, portable box which houses balanced spectrum fluorescent tubes. An individual's needs for light therapy specify the duration of exposure and the optimal time of day. An individual should meet periodically with a health care professional. The dose of light therapy can be adjusted as needed.

Who Suffers from SAD?

About 3/4 of SAD sufferers are women, but SAD affects men and children as well. The most typical age of onset is in the twenties, but other onsets are common, such as during puberty, middle age, and old age. After women pass through menopause, the numbers for men and women become equal. Susceptibility to SAD appears to be inherited. Fifty percent of fibromyalgia patients see a seasonal worsening of their symptoms.

The oldest form of light therapy is natural sunlight. The sun is the ultimate source of full-spectrum light, which means it contains all possible wavelengths of light, from infrared to ultraviolet (UV). Many forms of light therapy are now available, including full-spectrum light therapy, bright-light therapy, various forms of UV light therapy, syntonic optometry, cold laser therapy, and colored-light therapy. Electromagnetic devices, such as the Light Beam Generator and the MORA, also use specific light frequencies in treatment.

Turning the System on Untapped Abilities of the Mind

Ayurvedic Medicine

Ayurvedic Medicine categorizes the body into metabolic types. The goal of the treatment is to restore harmony of mind and spirit together with the environment. The term "Ayurvedic Medicine" means the "science of life."

Therapies use only natural methods to treat disease. Once the person's type is identified, then the treatment is prescribed. Treatment may be diet, exercise, yoga, meditation, massage, herbal tonics, herbal sweat baths, medicated enemas, and medicated inhalations.

The three body types are Vata, Pitta and Kapha. All three together are referred to as a Dosha. When the Doshas are balanced in accordance with an individual's constitution, the result is vibrant health and energy. Ayurvedic physicians have traditionally relied on the powers of observation rather than equipment and laboratory testing to diagnose disease. They observe their patients, asking questions about personal and family history, in addition to how the patient feels. They listen to the heart, lungs, and intestines. They examine the pulse, tongue, eyes, and nails, observing the tongue and urine for color and smell. After diagnosis, patients are placed into one of the four main methods of dealing with their conditions. Cleansing and detoxifying, palliation, rejuvenation, and hygiene are parts of the therapy.

Author's Opinion

This therapy must be administered by experts or at least people knowledgeable of the technology. Here again, the therapist becomes the detective searching for the cause, whether it be an enemy germ or other invader or an imbalance. This strategy is very good because it considers the powerful workings of the mind.

Voodoo

In the South Pacific and other less modern cultures is the religion of voodoo. The priest, called a witch doctor, teaches a young child the fears of disobeying the rules or falling out of favor with him. The witch doctor will make a doll as an image of a certain person. When this person does something wrong in the eyes of the witch doctor, he takes a needle and sticks it through the doll where the heart would be. The person, having been conditioned to believe that death is close, tenses up and with his mind and shuts down his body and dies. Death occurs within minutes.

I give this example to illustrate the power of the brain. There is no physical connection between the person and the doll.

The person who dies does so because of his or her belief. I know this for a fact because there have been times when someone did something wrong in the eyes of the witch doctor who was not completely indoctrinated.

In other words, the person doing the wrong did not believe in voodoo. The witch doctor dressed up a doll in the image of the person, built the fire for the ceremony, stuck the doll and nothing happened.

Your mind can bring you to instant ecstasy. Your mind can kill you in minutes. Do you recall my explanation of therapy in the example of the water circulating in pipes?

There are only a few reasons why water stops circulating through pipes. One is that the water itself is muddy and thick. Two is that the pipe could be crushed. Three is that someone shut the water off.

This "someone" who can shut the water off is the brain which can shut the body down causing it to die within minutes

Biofeedback

Biofeedback is a training program that teaches people how to change the rate of their heartbeat, as well as other automatic body functions. They use simple electronic devices.

Biofeedback is used to help minimize stress, headaches, asthmatic attacks, and pain. A person seeking to regulate his or her heart rate would train with a biofeedback device set up to transmit one blinking light or one audible beep per heartbeat.

By learning to alter the rate of the flashes and beeps, the subject is subtly programmed to control the heart rate.

Sleep disorders, hyperactivity in children and other behavioral disorders, dysfunctions stemming from inadequate control over muscles or muscle groups, incontinence, back pain, TMJ, and even loss of control due to brain or nerve damage have been improved through biofeedback.

It can also be used to treat heart dysfunction, gastrointestinal disorders, difficulty swallowing, esophageal dysfunction, ringing in the ears, twitching of the eyelids, fatigue, and cerebral palsy.

Author's Opinion

The ability to regulate one's heart rate is powerful. Many times a person gets an outside stimulation that triggers an attack--let's say a breathing attack. This sets other body responses in motion that otherwise would not happen. For example, a person has been told he has allergies; it is "allergy season," and a window is opened. The person begins to choke up. But there is no pollen in the breeze blowing in; the rag weed or golden rod are not yet to that stage. Yet the person has adverse reactions anyway.

Because this attack is "in the person's mind," methods such as biofeedback which deal with the mind are very successful in treating it. When this person had a mind-induced allergy attack, his focus was entirely on the attack. After he redirects his focus to regulating his heart rate, the allergy attack stops because the mind is no longer continuing it. What if you ate something and started to choke on it? Your body tenses up and you start to cough. When you are tense, the passages become smaller. Taking control of your breathing and heart rate would instantly relax you, and the passage would return to normal size. The object caught in your throat would then pass. I believe that it is very worthwhile to learn this technology. There are many books and papers written on biofeedback. Search for and read them. Direct your mind to focus on what you are looking for.

Neuro-Linguistic Programming

Neuro-Linguistic Programming (NLP) could be called "The Power of Positive Unconscious Thinking." It helps people detect and reprogram unconscious patterns of thought and behavior in order to alter psychological responses and enhance the healing process. NLP has been used with success for people suffering from nearly every condition imaginable.People who have difficulty recovering from physical illness have often adopted negative beliefs about their recovery. They perceive themselves as helpless, hopeless, worthless, and express thoughts like "I can't get healthy" or "There is no hope" or "I am not worth the effort." The primary goal of the NLP practitioner is to move a person from his or her present state of discomfort to a desired state of health and well-being by helping to reprogram beliefs about healing.

Benefits

By identifying and removing an individual's limiting belief about his or her condition, NLP has been shown to benefit a variety of health conditions and illnesses. Once these beliefs are redirected, the body is better able to utilize the immune system.

Author's Opinion

In my opinion, NLP is very worthwhile and merits further study. It deals with the mind's ability to control health. Do you remember the example of the water in the pipe? One of the reasons the water stops flowing is someone turned off the faucet, and the mind is like a person turning off a faucet. NLP shows the patient how to "turn it back on."

Guided Imagery

Guided Imagery is another method using the power of the mind to create a positive physical response. It is another player in the field of mind/body medicine. It has been used to reduce stress, slow heart rate, stimulate the immune system, and reduce pain. It is becoming more and more popular. When properly taught, it can also serve as a highly effective form of self-care.

The imagination is probably a person's least utilized health resource. It can be used to remember and recreate the past, develop insight into the present, influence physical health, enhance creativity and inspiration, and anticipate possible futures. Imagery is simply a flow of thoughts that one can see, hear, feel, smell, or taste in one's imagination. As an inner representation of experience, as well as fantasy, imagery is a rich, symbolic, and highly personal language. An image may or may not represent external reality, but it always represents internal reality. It is the language of the interface between mind and body.

It may seem difficult to believe that creating images in the mind can affect heart rate, lower blood pressure, restore respiratory patterns, affect oxygen consumption, facilitate carbon dioxide elimination, change brain wave rhythms, alter electrical characteristics of the skin, increase local blood flow and regulate the temperature of tissues, help gastrointestinal motility and secretions, create sexual arousal, regulate the levels of hormones and neurotransmitters in the blood, and immune system function. But it can, and the healing potentials of imagery go far beyond its remarkable ability to directly affect physiology. Imagery can be a key factor in dealing with either a simple tension headache or a life-threatening disease. It is a proven method for pain relief, for helping people tolerate medical procedures and treatments and reducing side-effects, and for stimulating healing responses in the body.

A person can change his or her attitude about anything using imaging. Changing your attitude leads to changing your emotions, and that leads to changing behaviors--and that leads to changing life-style patterns.

Whether the goal is to improve a medical condition, create more energy, or win a gold metal, imaging is a great addition to other treatment. Learning to relax is fundamental to self-healing, and imagery is a part of almost all relaxation and stress-reduction techniques. For many people, imagery is the easiest way to learn to relax, and its active nature makes it more comfortable than other methods of relaxation.

Meditation

It could be said that meditation is opposite of guided imagery. With guided imagery, the person is encouraged to create pictures in his or her mind of the future or the past. With meditation, the person is directed to a quiet focus on the present, focusing on breathing, and a certain image or a sound (mantra).

The person zooms in on aspects of this focus to quiet the mind to obtain clarity. It is a safe and simple way to balance a person's physical, emotional, and mental states. It is easily learned and has been used as an aid in treating stress and for pain management.

Many times meditation has been used as a part of other treatment strategies. The effectiveness depends on the person's ability to get his or her mind to focus on the present. Patients have been treated for stress management, hypertension, and heart disease.When the mind is calm and focused in the present, it is neither reacting to memories from the past, nor being preoccupied with plans for the future--two major sources of chronic stress known to impact health. Meditation helps to keep the patient from identifying with pictures in the mind which could trigger an emotional response that could cause stress and pain. This connection between the breath and one's state of mind is a basic principle of meditation.

Benefits

The benefits of meditation practice can be classified into three categories: physiological, psychological, and spiritual. In the category of physiology, meditative techniques have been used to promote health in the immune system, to treat cancer and AIDS, and to help allergies. In the category of psychology, these techniques are used to normalize brain rhythms and even control the body chemistry to help the patient get over alcohol, drug, and other addictions. It is taught to patients to help self-regulate disorders, such as anxiety, hypertension, and stress.

Sound Therapy

Certain sounds have been identified that can slow the breathing rate and create a feeling of overall well-being. Other sounds can slow a racing heart or soothe a restless baby. Sounds can also alter skin temperature, reduce blood pressure and muscle tension, and influence brain wave frequencies.

There is a direct connection between hearing impairment and vocal range, and a direct connection between hearing impairment and overall health and well-being. Sound therapy is used everywhere. People put music on without even knowing that they are employing sound therapy. Professionally it is used in hospitals, schools, corporate offices, and psychological treatment programs. They use it because it is a very effective addition to the treatment to reduce stress, lower blood pressure, alleviate pain, overcome learning disabilities, improve movement and balance, and promote endurance and strength.

The reason it is so effective is the ear is not only the primary organ of hearing, but it also has powerful influences on eye movement, rhythms of the physical body, prebirth brain growth, and general regulation of stress levels in the body.

Characteristic of this emerging field of Sound Therapy is the use of devices that utilize specific sound frequencies to achieve therapeutic benefits such as pain reduction or relaxation. Devices such as cymatic instruments and the Infratonic QGM are specific to sound therapy and being used worldwide.

Yoga

Yoga goes hand in hand with meditation because the focus is placed on the present. Like meditation, much attention is placed on breathing. It is one of the oldest known systems of health practiced in the world today. Research into yoga therapy has assured the people practicing it that it, in fact, does have scientific validity of therapeutic value. Yoga has had a strong impact on the fields of stress reduction, mind/body medicine, and energy medicine. Yoga is famous for the physical postures, breathing exercises, and meditation practices. It has been scientifically proven to reduce stress, lower blood pressure, regulate heart rate, and even retard the aging process.

The meaning of the word *yoga* is "union"--the integration of physical, mental, and spiritual energies that enhance health and well-being. Yoga teaches the main principle of mind/body unity. If the mind is chronically restless and agitated, the health of the body will be compromised, and if the body is in poor health, mental strength and clarity will be adversely affected. The practice of yoga can counter these ill effects, restoring mental and physical health.

Benefits

If a person is committed to yoga practice, the benefits can be enormous. These benefits are health, vitality, and peace of mind. Yoga was also shown to reduce both blood pressure and the need for drug therapy in patients suffering from hypertension.

Evaluating Any Therapy or Health Strategy

In evaluating any therapy or health strategy, one should ask and find answers for the following questions:

—Do I understand it?

—Is it logical? Are there parts of it that are not scientific?

—Does this therapy ask me to accept it without evidence?

—What are the risks?

—What is the stated effectiveness?

—What are my chances of receiving benefit?

—Is it easy to do?

—Can I afford it?

—Do I have the time?

—Does it fit my life-style?

—Do I like it? Is it for me?

Ongoing treatment is sometimes necessary and sometimes not. The challenge that we, the patients, have is knowing the difference. Therapists, like other business people, must pay bills, and continuous treatments provide cash flow.

When seeing any specialist or doctor, remember you have a right to ask questions. Ask your therapist if he or she will recommend some outside reading. Then read this information and verify that your treatment is correct and whether or not you actually need more than one treatment. Here is an example of abuse of therapy in the field of psychology. People used to go to psychologists for years and never get anywhere. Some would actually get worse as treatment continued.

About ten to twelve years ago, a young man, Anthony Robbins, without a college education, put these experts to shame. Robbins challenged these doctors to bring him their hardest-to-treat patients with the worst cases of phobia. Robbins would "treat" those patients right there over the phone or on stage in front of an audience. The treatments took less than thirty minutes, and the people were cured once and for all. People, for example, lost their fear of heights and snakes.

He gave (and still gives) one-stop therapy in getting rid of addictions along with strategies to condition the changes to become a natural way of life for the person. My person belief is that treatment from a specialist should take no more than four visits or five at most. The patients should learn to administer the treatment themselves and use the specialist as a coach. A coach should be available for questions and short treatment sessions. A coach is not a physician who assumes the role of the greatly feared witch doctor and will tell you nothing about your treatment.

As a thinking person, you cannot submit yourself fully to anyone. It is your body, and you must understand everything that is going on. You must be pro-active in the decision making process that involves your body, and you need to maintain an active role as the process continues.

There are thousands of health strategies. You cannot become an expert in them all, though it would be nice. Then you could select your strategy from a real position of knowledge. Every one of these health strategies has some merit, and eventually there should arise people who become experts in them all.

Unfortunately, the keen minds of many qualified people are wasted doing research and experiments in search of a better antibiotic. They waste their time and talents doing detective work that will never take them anywhere except a blind alley. You, as an individual, are capable of that kind of knowledge, and you can dedicate your life to it.

How much time do you spend watching television? If you spent just half that time studying, you could learn great things about alternative choices that could provide you with a healthier life.

If your time must be spent earning a living and taking care of other responsibilities, you, at least, need to know how to evaluate these strategies. You need to know what is safe and effective as well as what is harmful.

Chapter Two

You Are the Doctor

When the experts depart from science, it's time to depart from the experts. There seems to be arising a whole industry of people who mean very well, and who wish to do good, but these people are people just like everyone else. The problem is some think they have a monopoly over medicine (and other things). They think they are the only ones who are smart enough to figure things out and prescribe what is good for the rest of us. I believe all people are basically the same, including these people. They did not put themselves in this position of adoration--we put them there. Some patients are so thankful for their doctors and adore them so much that their admiration is almost worship. As a culture, we adore and worship a lot of people in other areas as well, such as sports, religion, and entertainment. This idol worship syndrome has become part of the fabric of America's thinking, and it can have a negative side. Too much idol worship leads us to be dependent upon other people to solve all of life's problems. We then don't work to solve our own problems.

This idol worship mindset is not in and of itself all bad. It has worked for several years and may still work in certain areas. But when medical mistakes are common, the cost of letting other people take this responsibility becomes too high. You entrust your body to the care of a doctor, and he or she makes decisions without consulting you. Whether the decisions are correct or not, you are still ultimately responsible, yet you had no part in making those decisions. In no area of business do you make agreements and contracts like this. Your health and life are far too important to continue to make these contracts. You must remember that it is your body, and you stand to lose, or gain. You must take control. You must become your own doctor. The expert to whom you go, your doctor, must be your advisor. You must quit being a submissive sufferer (a patient).

This chapter is dedicated to those of you who are ready to take on that responsibility. First, here is some interesting information you need to know. The human body is an incredible masterpiece. It travels through processes called aging. While our desires, needs, and health requirements are different as we age, there are basic things common to all. There are certain health rules we can break and still be healthy. There are certain rules we cannot break. Among these rules, some are more important than others. When you look for the way to operate a car, for example, you look in the manufacturer's manual. It is the manufacturer who has laid out the design and intended that a certain fuel be used, and so on. You would never put diesel in a gas engine. Likewise, the human body has a manual, a guide. For operational instructions you turn to the manufacturer's manual—the Bible.

According to the Bible, we were made from the dust of the earth. Therefore, our body must be nourished with every single mineral or element found in the earth. Because plants that we eat grow out of the earth, and animals eat plants that grow out of the earth, these minerals should be found in the plants and animals we eat. Whether or not this is so is debatable.

When I hear it said that our soil doesn't contain these nutrients,

I recall a Law of Thermodynamics. "Nothing is created. Nothing is destroyed." Water evaporates and returns in the form of dew and rain. Minerals travel into plants and return when the plant dies and decays. While I do not necessarily disagree, I personally do not believe our food is completely void of nutrients. I believe the problem is over processing, and our personal food choices are more the culprit than the foods themselves.

These rules are few, and very simple. Eat animals that have a cloven (divided) hoof and chew their cud. Animals with paws or claws do not qualify. Of the animals that live in the water, eat only those that have scales and fins. Shellfish do not qualify. Of the animals that fly, eat only those that are not scavengers. It's OK to eat insects from the locust, beetle, and grasshopper families. Anyone who knows these rules can select healthy food to eat. You don't have to do a laboratory analysis of nutrient content. All you have to do is to be able to see that animal. Does this fish have scales and fins? Does this animal chew its cud and have a cloven hoof? It's easy. Anyone can do it.

Pay close attention to meat that is left over a period of 24 hours. The second an animal dies, it starts to decay. This breaking down process is the process of returning living things to the dust of the earth. There are microscopic plants and animals that assist in this process. Food stored too long is loaded with these little guys. It is said that the environment is polluted. Fish in polluted water are not fit to eat. Animals grazing on radiated grasses are somehow altered. But if we keep these simple rules stated above, we don't have to be careful of the diet of these animals. Why? Because these animals have a purification system. For example, cows have four stomachs. Everything they eat goes through a long digestive process. Pigs, on the other hand, do not. Food that pigs eat goes onto their body as meat within four hours. Fish with scales and fins have a purification system to keep poisons from going into their muscles. If you found a fish with scales and fins swimming in raw sewage, it is only common sense that you should not eat it. The rules of common sense are always in effect.

The point I am making is that in spite of the horror stories we hear about our polluted food supply, the facts are that we eat these foods day after day and stay healthy. While there are exceptions, the evidence does not support the assertions that our food supply is as polluted as some say. There are also rules that cannot be violated regarding eating these clean animals. These rules are simple.

Do not eat blood, fat, or any organs that are for cleansing such as the intestines or kidneys. Why? Because the blood is a transportation system, ridding the body of poisons. Fat is a storage place for excessive poisons that the body cannot eliminate. Cleansing organs are concentrated with the poisons that have been collected.

The accounts of the lives of people in Biblical times tell us that they were busy working. They did not have the time to do what it would take to kill and eat an animal. They did not have refrigeration, so they could not properly store leftovers. Therefore, they ate fresh fruit and vegetables. Then, on days of rest and holidays, or when they were celebrating, they ate meat, drank wine or strong drink, and ate bread. They only ate these things when they had time to relax and allow their body to take the extra energy it needed to digest the feast.

When they needed to work, they didn't overload their bodies with meat or strong drink. The key is common sense and moderation. Another key health rule is simple. Pay attention to the weekly cycle. There are seven days. Work six of these days and rest one. Violating this rule creates mental anguish and turmoil. We call it stress or burn out. In my own life I have tried it both ways. I have noticed that I can get more done in six days than I can in seven because the work I do in the six days is relatively mistake free since I am better focused.

When someone becomes infected with a contagious disease, that person is isolated from the rest of society. Why? Not because germs would spread, but because the poison would spread. The next logical question is, how do you know if a person has a contagious disease? If he or she is eliminating poisons. These poisons can come through the nose, mouth, skin, or the large or small intestines. These poisons are found in blood, saliva, phlegm, and pus, to name a few. You can tell a person has a contagious disease because you can see and smell the poison.

When a person touches a dead human body or the dead body of an animal that was not intended to be eaten, the person should stay away from other people for the rest of the day. Why? Because when an animal or person dies, the individual or animal loses its osmotic pressure. This means their intestines, bladder, and other organs no longer have muscle strength to hold their substances. Poisons from this dead body may be transmitted to the person handling them. These poisons take several hours to dissipate and thus should not be spread to other people.

If any poisonous bodily fluid touches anything, the things it touches are contaminated and should be thrown away or destroyed. Exceptions to this would be very nonporous materials, such as glass or stainless steel.

You must work and you must sweat, though it be ever so slightly. Sweat flushes poisons out of the body. These are poisons that cannot be disposed of in any other way.

Another rule from the Bible that you cannot violate and still have good health is this: You must not allow your mind to delve in negativity, but you must focus on positive things. "Whatsoever things are true, whatsoever things are honest, whatsoever things are just, whatsoever things are pure, whatsoever things are lovely, whatsoever things are of good report; if there be any virtue and if there be any praise, think on these things." *Philippians 4:8.* To become your own doctor, you need to be aware of the tools that are available. (Please refer to the chapter on alternative strategies.)

Of these strategies, there is none so effective or risk free as magnetic therapy. If you apply the rules of logic and common sense, magnetic therapy is the first place to start.

How To Work with Magnetic Therapy

I have organized this therapy by the kind of magnet and the way to use it. We are assuming that all of these magnets are properly designed for the purposes of health improvement. There are two kinds of therapeutic magnets.

1) A magnet with one pole on each surface.

2) Lodestone-type magnets that are referred to as natural magnetism without attention to pole placement.

First, we will discuss the applications for the first division, magnets with one pole on each surface. This is also refereed to as uni-pole. *Uni* means *one*. *Uni-pole* means *one pole on each surface.*

Treat the Symptoms

Place the north pole of a properly designed therapeutic magnetic product directly over the symptom. It can be skin eruptions, muscle or joint pain, lumps, whether it is calcium buildup or disorganized tissue, a parasite such as a wart, an injury, burns, muscle tremors, and any kind of soreness or other symptom.

Pain from Recent Injuries

The most dramatic demonstration of the effectiveness of magnetic therapy is placing the north pole directly over a burn, bump, or cut. If the injury is recent—within the first minute—cover the entire injury with the magnet, and the pain can go away in seconds. This happens because all injuries have one thing in common—energy out of balance. Let's discuss this issue.

There are five energy variables: frequency, power, pole, pattern, and ability to penetrate. Of these five characteristics, which one do you think is responsible for this imbalance? Let us consider these one by one.

Recall the spiraling force field. The frequency is the speed of the spin. The power is the size of the circle. The pole is the direction of the spin, either clockwise or counter-clockwise. The pattern is force fields coming from two or more different sources to create a specific pattern. The ability to pentetrate is the intensity of the force field and depends on the size of the magnet.

Could it be frequency? Sensitive instruments that measure frequency can measure different frequencies all over the body. There is no balancing requirement. So frequency is probably not the problem.

Could it be power? Yes, it is possible. But think about it. You slam your finger in the car door. The pain is excruciating. The body is a generator of power, and it is logical to assume that this painful area is emitting a higher power. How can you turn the power down on an injury? Power is another characteristic that is not balanced within a single force field. Let's rule out power.

Could it be the energy pattern? Remember, this energy pattern is a pattern of poles. There are only two choices: All one pole or alternating poles. We know it cannot be alternating poles because this does not occur naturally in nature. Energy sources all emit equal energy from both poles, but they do it on one side at a time. Alternating is an invention of man as a method to get electricity to travel greater distances. So we can eliminate energy pattern.

Could it be the ability to penetrate? Here again it is not logical. Your finger is in excruciating pain. This extra energy at the site is bursting out on all sides. You cannot do anything about the penetrating inward. It is not logical to try to shield the penetration outward in an attempt to balance it. We rule out this characteristic.

The only other choice we have is the direction of the spin, referred to as the pole. There must be equal amounts (balance) of energy from both poles. Instruments measure greater south pole energy at the site of injuries than north pole energy. Of the five choices, this is the only one we can do anything about. We can overpower the excessive south pole energy with more powerful north pole energy.

I probably burn myself at least a couple of times a year, generally on a stove. I keep a magnet nearby and use it. I put the north pole of the magnet directly over the burn, and the pain goes away in seconds. Sometimes the burn is bad enough for the pain to come back.

Then I put the magnet right back over it, and the pain is gone again in a few seconds. It never blisters, peels, or hurts anymore. Sometimes I will tape the magnet over the burn for added insurance.

Let's summarize: You burn your hand. Place the north pole of a properly designed therapeutic magnet directly over the burn. The pain goes away in seconds.

Why? Because at the site of this symptom, there is excessive south pole energy. How do we know? Because instruments can measure it. One example is the MRI. Its operation is simple. It scans the body searching for excessive south pole energy. It sends signals to a computer and the computer displays it on the screen.

The only "things" the person who looks at this picture can see are the places where there is excessive south pole energy. The doctor will ask the patient about their symptoms and piece together other details to determine the real problem.

Another way we know about energy healing is with a simple test. We have an area with excessive south pole energy. To restore balance, we give that area more powerful, north pole energy. The evidence that balance is restored is a change in the intensity of the symptoms. Bright redness will become pink, pain will recede, acid will be neutralized, and, as a result, the irritation will diminish.

When you place the more powerful force field of north pole energy directly at the site, you are restoring the energy balance. This instantly corrects the chaos caused by the hot surface. It instantly starts repairing the cells.

It is just that simple. The counterclockwise spinning energy of a properly designed therapeutic magnet restores. Do you understand why it is so important to use a properly designed therapeutic magnet?

It can work with every person every time. Skeptical people will not admit they were even hurt in the first place, or they will say the injury was not that bad. These people are not ready to learn because they don't have the courage to face the responsibility of becoming their own doctor. They are not ready to take charge of their health.

Tumors or Disorganized, Unnatural Growths

For tumors, place the north pole of a properly designed

therapeutic magnet directly over the growth. If the growth is internal, place the magnet over it from the outside. Although you cannot see exactly where the growth is, be as precise as possible. Ask your doctor to show you where the growth is located. If there are a number of growths, then cover the entire area with magnets. How does it work? Why does it happen? Let's direct our explanation to the smallest units, the cells. Think about a tornado hitting a house. Think about the magnet's energy following and putting it back together again. It happens in this case, too. But in the case of badly disorganized cells, it takes more than that.

Think again of the house that is destroyed by a tornado and what happens after it lies for years and years. What if the stronger, more powerful reverse force field of the magnet hit it? What would happen? Not much. Why? Because the lumber, rotted and decayed, is at a point of no return. If you are going to restore this house, you need new materials. It is the same with the cells of so-called cancerous tumors. A good example of what the cells in this tumor look like is corn smelt. These gray, ugly kernels of corn grow up out of the ear in all directions. They are soft, and they smell. Some are long and curly; others have their skin broken open, oozing out fluid.

The strategy to eliminate disorganized growth is to replace each cell with good, strong, healthy ones. The brain does this naturally without any help from us, except we need to live a life-style in which proper oxygen and nutrients are supplied to the cell. When cells have ample oxygen and nutrients, and have the circulatory ability to carry away the waste, then strong, healthy cells are produced.

These strong, healthy cells replace the ugly, disorganized ones. It is just that simple. The reason we have disorganized cells in the first place is because the transportation of oxygen and nutrients is slowed down or cut off.

The out-going transportation of waste products is also slowed down or cut off. The cell drowns in its own waste and doesn't have the supplies to repair itself or to do anything about it. Do your part to restore circulation, and the turnaround is immediate.

I have seen sores that were called skin cancer respond to improved circulation within twenty minutes of being exposed to a magnet. This same sore started to diminish in four days. By the end of the week, it was gone. People do not need to die from this epidemic. Isn't it a shame that everyone doesn't know about this? The use of magnets is so simple, so effective, and so safe and underrated.

Parasite Symptoms

When we think of "parasites," most people think of "worms." But parasites are more than just worms. There are thousands of plants and animals feeding in and on our bodies as they devour poisons. These are our friends, hauling away the garbage just like scavengers clean the bottom of rivers and lakes.

The Bible organizes animals and plants according to whether or not the being is a parasite or not. If a parasite, it is called "unclean." There is nothing more logical than the practice of eating clean animals and not unclean animals. If an animal instinctively eats poisons, by way of keeping the earth clean, then some of those poisons are going to stay in its body. It is just plain stupid to eat poison. That is what you are doing if you eat these animals.

While there are some parasites in the body big enough to see, there are millions of others that are microscopic. These little guys eat little particles of waste too small for worms. And, they eat the waste products left by the worms and other parasites.

From time to time, parasite activity becomes a symptom,

appearing as a skin rash. If you look at your blood under a microscope, you can see them. They may even be painful. These symptoms are a signal of poor circulation.

How do we know? Because parasites, germs, yeast, molds, or fungus, just to name a few, do not feed on healthy tissue. They only feed on decay and poison. If there is no poison or decay present, there will be no parasites.

If the body's transportation system is flowing freely, poisons are being flushed away through proper channels. If not, poisons start to collect, slow circulation, and create pressure at the site. Sometimes this pressure is so great it pushes them right through the pores of the skin. As it pushes through the skin, it damages the cells and sometimes causes bleeding. Doctors call this condition eczema, or psoriasis. We call it a rash. If you place a magnet directly over it, the spinning force fields will cause the slow, circulating molecules to spin, causing the cells to vibrate, and the poisons will start to move out. The pressure will be reduced. The poison will stop oozing through the skin, and the rash goes away.

You should not use antibiotics to kill parasites. In fact, if you are successful at killing them all, more resilient strains of parasites that you cannot kill will appear. If you have a skin rash, you don't have a skin problem or a parasite problem. You have a circulation problem. There is nothing more effective than a magnet to improve circulation directly at the site. Most parasites thrive in a low-oxygen, low-pH environment. Properly designed, therapeutic magnets can restore circulation, deliver oxygen to the site, and rearrange hydrogen molecules to raise pH, and the parasites that live in an acid environment die.

Muscle or Joint Pain

For muscle or joint pain, place the magnet directly over the painful area. As far as magnetic therapy is concerned, it doesn't matter what the cause is. It may completely solve the problem. It may happen with your first exposure to the magnet. It may take several days, weeks, or months.

If the same problem reoccurs, you should conduct an investigation to find the cause. Take this investigation seriously. Keep records. Keep a journal. If you are going to become your own doctor, you must keep records.

If you don't find the cause, the resulting pain will continue, and you can always use the magnet. Magnets relieve pain, but the present technology in magnetic therapy is cumbersome and clumsy. In some cases, you have to strap a huge magnet to your body. You have to sleep with this strapped in place.

To make yourself go to this extra trouble, you must be very motivated. Sleeping with "rocks" is not easy. During the day, people will look at you and make you feel like you are crazy. You will not continue unless you are very motivated. This is why you need to know how and why magnets work.

And, you need to understand that they do, indeed, work. If you don't absolutely believe and understand that they will work, the ridicule and discomfort will not be worth it.

The following is an attempt to identify some causes for pain. This list is by no means complete, although, I have done my best to consider them all.

Structural

The origination of the problem is probably lower in your body. Think about the foundation of a house. Imagine that the foundation drops down on one corner. A chain reaction happens throughout the rest of the house. You can repair a wall here and a floor there, but unless you repair the foundation, the wall and floor will need repair again because there is constant pressure throwing them off. If you believe this is your predicament, you have a couple of choices.

One would be wise to have an expert such as a chiropractor look at your body and physically put it back into place. There are problems that these people, and only these people, can solve. Then there are other problems that they try to solve, but they are never quite successful at solving. If this is the case with you, will never quit going for your adjustment. Your treatment will give you relief for a short while, but the pain will return.

It is just like using a magnet, only more expensive. To get relief, the treatment must be a way of life. However, treatments were not meant to be ways of life. God intended life to be active and pain free. When the pain originates somewhere else, the real cause may be hard to find, but if you are committed to finding it, you will.

Another treatment choice most may not be familiar with is the Egoscue Method. According to Pete Egoscue, your body was designed to last at least a hundred years. Elderly people should be able to work like they did when they were in their forties. They should be able to swim and run and do whatever they want. There is no reason to suffer with diseases of aging. There is no such thing.

If your muscles or joints hurt, there is a fixable reason. If the reason is structural, it means foundation muscles are too weak to support your structure. Your body could be compared with a house that has a weak foundation. The integrity of every part of the house is compromised. To solve this problem, you must repair the foundation first, then the rest of the house.

The strategy behind The Egoscue Method is fixing the foundation. Pete Egoscue can look at a person's posture and tell which muscles are weak. He designs gentle, easy exercises to strengthen these muscles.

For further information, please see his two books *The Egoscue Method of Health Through Motion* and *Pain Free a Revolutionary Method for Stopping Chronic Pain.* If circumstances permit, call his clinic in San Diego, California. His entire staff is trained to duplicate his work. They respect you in your role of being your own doctor. I am one of his clients.

I have had pain in my jaw my entire life, and my left knee clicks and hurts when I walk. I suffer from chronic headaches, and I have had searing, hot pain between my shoulder blades. The way I coped with the pain in my jaw was to have my dentist grind off certain surfaces on my teeth for a better bite. It was somewhat successful but really wasn't the answer. Eating a simple salad was still painful. To live with the pain between my shoulder blades, I position a large therapeutic magnet there every time I sit. It works. The pain goes away in seconds, and as long as the magnet is in place, there is no pain. It stays gone for a few hours then comes back. To solve the problem of clicking and pain in my knee, I try not to use it, but when I must be on my feet for hours at a time, it hurts a lot.

Pete does not buy the diagnosis of pain and problems being inherited and, therefore, impossible to solve. In other words, he does not believe we are harnessed by inherited conditions we can do nothing about.

Our bodies were not made for a life of pain. The therapist at his clinic says my structure is not straight and my brain's delivery of oxygen is cut off. My headaches are the results of the brain screaming for oxygen. To solve this problem, I have been using magnets. I sleep in a magnetic cap. A friend of mine offered another magnetic solution, and that is putting magnets in my ears over acupuncture points. The force fields open congested electrical highways. This assists the delivery of oxygen to the brain and my headaches disappear.

At the time of this writing, I have been doing the exercises in the Egoscue Method every morning for about two months. Every one of these problems is being solved. I still have them, but not as severe. Why does this work? It works because the exercises are strengthening foundation muscles that are supposed to support the bone structure. When the muscles intended to support it do not properly support the structure, other muscles step in to compensate. These "good will" muscles quickly become overworked. They were not designed for that particular task. Strengthen the foundation of the body, and the body rebuilds itself.

When I first started these exercises, my body was stiff. My prescribed program was gentle, yet it was quite challenging for me. Magnets again came to the rescue. I placed magnets on these stiff muscles during the exercises. Almost immediately, I could feel the energy transfer from the magnet to me. The stiff muscles loosened up, and I did the exercises with ease. I only had to use the magnets once. These little used, stiff muscles responded in one exercise session.

As the blessing of technology makes our lives easier and easier, we find ourselves less and less active. When we don't use our muscles, we lose them. If our foundation muscles become so weak that they no longer support our structure, we will have pain. Magnetic therapy in this case is a first-aid strategy but does not solve the real problem. The only real answer is to strengthen the foundation muscles.

Damage from Outside Force Fields

Imaginations and paranoia run amuck. Sometimes we invent things to fear. There's an old saying to try to soothe the nerves of those of us who see false danger everywhere. "What you don't see can't hurt you." The problem with that statement is that it is true only some of the time. If you spend time in a building that has electricity or near any kind of electrical appliance or electrical wire, dangerous force fields are bombarding and penetrating your body. This is just one of the examples of things you don't see that can hurt you. See the chapter in this book entitled "Harmful Force Fields" for a complete discussion of this subject.

We are creatures of habit. We get up at the same time every morning. We eat basically the same things day after day. We think the same things over and over. The culture we live in is unprecedented. Never before in the history of the world have people lived in such luxury. People living at the so-called poverty level are more comfortable than kings were 60 years ago.

The biggest reason for this huge rise in quality life-style is because of electricity. With the flip of a switch, an entire football field is as light as day, information is delivered to us from the other side of the world, our carpet is cleaned, our food is cooked, and our hair is dry. Every challenge the inventors and engineers had with electricity has been solved: cost, fire hazard, distribution, that is, except one. Its force fields are bombarding us, disrupting our cells, and causing stress and damage to our bodies.

As a result, the body has extra damage to repair, which reduces its energy. When the body's energy is no longer strong enough to repair, this damages individual cells and causes them to grow chaotically. These cells can no longer do their work. These body team members, who used to do their part, become useless to the body and are in the way. Their buildup causes circulation to be restricted. Oxygen is no longer delivered, nor are nutrients. Waste products build up and pH lowers. Parasites, the body's cleaning crew, move in to clean up the "garbage." As the condition worsens, the body sends a signal of pain.

If these force fields bombard organs, they can no longer function at peak efficiency. When they can no longer do their job, other organs try to help. Because these compensating organs are now doing extra work, like any other muscle that is exercised, they get bigger, and pressure develops. This scenario could go on forever. Far too many diseases and health problems are misdiagnosed because the person who diagnosed them did not consider these dangerous force fields. The treatment for this problem is very simple. First of all, it would be a good idea to figure out where the force fields are hitting you. Here again you must conduct a structured investigation. Any good detective would jump at the opportunity to solve such an easy problem. Your investigation is a mere process of elimination.

Start with your morning and write down every place you spend 30 or more minutes in each day. You can narrow the search by considering any place in your body where there is pain. Look for the obvious. Then ask yourself questions to determine where you spend time that has potentially dangerous force fields that could be penetrating your body. If your problem is throughout the entire body, look for bodily exposure such as from an electric blanket or an electrically heated waterbed. As stated above, find the force fields bombarding you and do something about them. Figure out a way to shield yourself from them. Increase your distance from appliances and televisions sets whenever possible.

Malfunctioning Organs

There are a lot of reasons for malfunctioning organs, but with magnetic therapy, the reasons really shouldn't concern us. What matters are the changes we make to our life-style so the damage doesn't progress or worsen. To solve this problem, it is necessary to know more about our organs and how they work. You need to know what happens and what symptoms the body manifests when these organs are not working.

For example, if you have low blood sugar, the problem is probably your pancreas. People have told me they placed a large penetrating magnet directly over their pancreas, took their blood sugar level before and after the treatment, and their blood sugar level was lower in twenty minutes. It doesn't matter which organ one is treating.

The reason magnetic therapy works is basically the same. Circulation is increased; therefore, the organ is getting the supplies and building blocks it needs to do its job. There is a transfer of energy. Organs are muscles. Weak muscles need more strength. The immediate transfer of increased energy from a therapeutic magnet is about thirty percent. This is easily demonstrated. Do a strength test. Write down the results. Stand on a magnet or magnets while doing the same strength test. The results can be about thirty percent better.

This test is done with south pole or alternating energy. Never use south pole energy for therapeutic reasons. Dr. Davis and Dr. Rawls tried it and found it caused lab animals to age prematurely. The only variable that is changed to determine if energy is north or south is the direction of the spin. North pole energy is healing energy. South pole energy is energizing energy.

High or low blood pressure could be symptoms of a sluggish organ. There are three basic strategies. One is to wear a magnetic necklace or chain around your neck six days out of the week. The second is to hold a magnet in your right hand, put a blood pressure cuff on your arm, and watch the blood pressure go to normal. The third is to identify the sluggish organ and place a large penetrating magnet there.

Eye Disorders

Many eye disorders result from poor circulation, which is not surprising considering the blood vessels in the eye area are very tiny. Because circulation is a major problem, magnetic therapy is successful. The retina degenerates with age, and the person becomes blind. But this doesn't happen to everyone, only those who have poor circulation in that area. The retina degenerates because it is not getting enough oxygen or nutrients. Waste products get stuck in the tiny pathways. The cells are not only starved, but also wallow in their own waste. They deteriorate quickly.

Place a properly designed force field from a magnet directly over the eye area. The penetrating force fields condition the blood and tissue making individual components smaller so they circulate better. Right away the cells are supplied with what they need to do their job. In very short order, the cells in the retina are restored and the person's sight problems are over. I have seen this demonstrated over and over again. The first time was about three years ago when we received a call from a man whose mother was legally blind. She could not do her housework. She could not read her mail. Her son helped her get the right magnets to place over the eyes and the area around the eyes. She slept with them in place at night, and within six weeks, this eighty-six-year-old woman was seeing again. It completely changed her life.

Whenever you place magnets over an area of extremely poor circulation, the poisons move out quickly. If a person is exposed to excessive poisons, there are symptoms. These symptoms in the eye area are usually burning sensations. These symptoms also happen when the poisons move out. If you understand this, and even expect it, you will not be alarmed.

But if you don't understand it, you may think the magnets are hurting you. These adverse symptoms are only temporary. There is only so much poison and toxin buildup. When it is gone, the symptoms will cease. With the poisons gone and the supplies provided to the cells adequate, the cells have what they need to function and reproduce, replacing the deteriorated ones. Other eye disorders are caused by misplaced tissue build up that covers the retina. We will discuss this in the next subsection about tissue build up.

Scar Tissue Buildup

Have you ever watched a stream from day to day? If you have, you've noticed a change in its path. Debris falls into the water that is too big to float away and collects on one side of the stream. The water makes a path around it. Sometimes the debris is so much it stops the flow of the water completely. A pond or waterfall results. Imagine debris collecting in the body's circulatory system, collecting on the side of the vessels. As debris builds up in a stream, tissue builds up in places other than its intended area. This tissue mass sometimes covers the retina. These are called cataracts. The body's master system that regulates new cell growth, responds very quickly when magnets are placed directly over this area.

When your skin is cut, the cells at the site react quickly to repair the damage. They close the area as fast as possible. Unfortunately, they do the job a little too quickly. They reproduce so quickly that the result is unnecessary tissue. This is referred to as scar tissue. There have been cases in which the scar tissue closed off circulating electrical signals from the brain to the rest of the body, therefore, paralyzing the person.

Pain Caused by Calcium Buildup

Calcium buildup can sometimes be seen as bumps sticking through the skin. It can build up on the hands so severely that they become stiff and frozen. Sometimes calcium build up is called a bone or heal spur. Getting rid of the excess build up is easy for magnets. In fact, you can see the collapsing of the actual calcium molecule under a

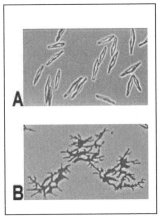

microscope. In this picture, we focused in on the calcium molecule. We took this picture and then passed a magnet over it and took another picture. In the first picture, the calcium looks like a feather or a snowflake. Because all force fields travel in circles, this spinning action causes this calcium molecule to spin. As it spins, the rough edges are removed, and it becomes streamlined. Now this streamlined calcium molecule can circulate through the blood stream better. There is nothing for it to stick to. If there had been an electrical charge to cause it to stick to the bone, the magnetic field neutralizes this charge, too.

Step one is accomplished, which is stopping further build up of more calcium. Next, the lump needs to be broken. As the spinning force fields penetrate it, they chip away at it one molecule at a time. Over the next few weeks, most lumps are well on their way toward disappearing.

If wanting to rid the hands of calcium build up, magnetic placement is a little more complicated. To my knowledge, there is no such thing as a magnetic glove. I have seen partial gloves with half fingers, but the magnets in these gloves were so small the energy would not penetrate with enough power to do any good. While it is always best to place magnets directly over symptoms, this is impractical when working with areas such as hands. The next best thing is a magnetic wrist wrap or bracelet. There are a number of reasons why this procedure works.

All the blood that travels through the hand must first go through the wrist. Therefore, the calcium in the blood is delivered in a conditioned, streamlined state.

The calcified lumps do not get the benefits of direct force fields, but the blood cells become magnetized by passing through the force field from the wrist wrap or bracelet to penetrate and dissolve them. I have seen hands that had been stiff, painful, and frozen for several years become young and limber again.

Addictions

Dr. William Philpott states in the book *Biomagnetic Handbook* "Addiction is a state in which a drug, food, or chemical containing a narcotic (exorphin) produces a pleasurable brain reaction, relieves physical symptoms and, in general, soothes both physically and emotionally. In addition, frequently-used foods and chemicals can evoke the body to produce self-made narcotics (endorphins). When endorphin production exceeds the body's physiological need for endorphins, they become as addicting as exorphins." So, the body is getting endorphins in the form of exorphins. To keep the system from this damage, the body's natural endorphin producers shut down. With the endorphin producers shut down, the body must get this sense of pleasure, pain relief, and soothing from outside sources.

When the person wants to be free from the substance, he or she endures the traumatic, stressful feelings until the body's natural endorphin producers begin to function again. Excessive south pole energy is stimulating and overdriving the brain and body causing the entire body to be out of balance.

In this case, when the body is out of balance, it is because there is excessive south pole energy. To restore balance, the energy of the north pole of a magnet will help. Place a large therapeutic magnet over the lungs, and within five minutes or less your craving can cease. For example, if you had wanted a cigarette, you may not want it. To reduce anxiety attacks, place the proper magnet directly over the temples. Anxiety attacks may subside. You can use this treatment more than once.

Eventually, the endorphin producers will be back in full swing and, except in the person's desire for them, they will not physically need the substance for a sense of well being.

Other magnetic treatments that have helped people break addictions are sleeping on a properly designed therapeutic mattress pad, sleeping with extra magnets on their head—as in a magnetic cap—and placing the proper magnet directly over the area in which symptoms are found.

Acupuncture with Magnets Instead of Needles

The objective of acupuncture is to deliver energy to the site of the injury. Acupuncture works through the body's large network of electrical connections. Electrical signals are supposed to circulate freely. When they get obstructed, the body develops adverse symptoms.

When this electrical highway circulates freely, the adverse symptoms depart. The junction where the highway crosses is called an acupuncture point. The place where the symptoms develop tells the acupuncturist where to perform the therapy.

The therapy is performed by piercing the body with little needles. Because the body is slightly injured, it feels an immediate burst of energy. This energy is supposed to move quickly through the electrical highway and clear pathway.

When the highway is clear, and the signals can pass, the symptoms should disappear. If they don't, the acupuncturist will select another acupuncture point to insert more needles.

You can do the same thing with acupuncture point magnets. To be considered an acupuncture point magnet, the magnet must be round and no larger that nine millimeters. The energy from the magnet penetrates the body and finds the electrical highway. It travels down it to clear it out.

To clear up symptoms, you must find the right point or points and the highway must, in fact, have been obstructed in the first place. A breathing disease can be successfully treated by using the acupuncture points at each side of the nose, placed in the lower corners.

Natural Magnetism

I hear of and meet people all the time who say they have been using magnets for health reasons for twenty-five and sometimes even forty years. While the popular wisdom regarding how magnets work is that no one really knows how it works, this book proves that statement to be false. We know how magnets work and why they work. When magnetic force fields penetrate the body, many things can happen. We choose the easiest way to understand concepts and to explain how and why they work. When I ask where these people got their magnets and how they knew one magnet from another, they answered that it was pretty much hit or miss. If the injury didn't respond, they tried a different magnet. They didn't know the difference between the north and the south pole. From time to time, that actually caused injuries to get worse. So, how do you know what is a properly designed therapeutic magnet and what is not? You should start by biting the bullet and spending a little more money to purchase the magnet from a company that knows magnets.

Make sure the salesperson understands how and why they work. Make sure they are not bi-polar or alternating. A good question to ask is: "Does it matter which side I place next to my body?" If it doesn't matter, then both poles are present on both sides. This is bi-polar or alternating. If it does matter, then the north pole is on one side, and the south pole is on the other. This is the kind you want. There is an exception to this rule. When using magnetic acupuncture, it doesn't matter because your goal is to move energy through the highway. Either pole will accomplish this movement.

I have a question for you: "Which is better, the old or the new?" The answer is that it doesn't matter. While we would most likely choose the old, it is not necessarily the best. We assume the old is better because we assume more people have been using it. Perhaps we assume this gold mine has been hidden all these years, and now it is discovered. If true, then we could assume that the old is better because there has been more experience with the tried and true. However, technology has proven all of these assumptions to be false. For example, is the typewriter or the word processor better? The carburetor or the fuel injector? An insulated box you put ice in or the refrigerator? In each example, the new is better.

Magnetic technology is no exception, but the truth of the matter is that the age-old, tried and true, magnetic technology is not alternating. It is natural magnetism.

What is the difference? With alternating, the poles are precisely placed on the magnet to create a pattern of north and south pole energy. This pattern can be seen in iron filings. Magnetizers are so advanced today that they can produce virtually any pattern— straight lines, checkerboard, triangles, or they can draw pictures.

Natural magnetism, on the other hand, has no attention to pole placement. Lodestone is an example. It was a lodestone that was fashioned into the piece of forehead jewelry that Cleopatra was famous for. Cleopatra wore the lodestone in the middle of her forehead to improve circulation to her face, and maybe even the rest of her body.

Her strategy was acupuncture. In the middle of the forehead is a main acupuncture point. It is so important and well known that it even has a name--*The Third Eye*.

Placing the magnet directly on the acupuncture point assured the delivery of oxygen and nutrients to her face. Did it work? According to some historians, her beauty was legendary. The one thing that creates, maintains, and restores beauty is circulation. The skin, hair, and nails must have oxygen, nutrients, and must get rid of poisons. To have real beauty, circulation is absolutely essential. In fact, most beauty treatments have the same goal—improve circulation.

Now, after Davis and Rawls discovered the difference in the energy between the north and the south poles, we have even better tools than Cleopatra's. When someone refers to magnetic therapy as being 4,000 years old, they are referring to natural magnetism, without attention to pole placement. Alternating technology is probably as old as the advent of the magnetizer. All north pole magnetism is about forty years old. As mentioned above, natural magnetism is very effective in the treatment of blood pressure.

While third world cultures are still using raw lodestone with some success, it is not the best strategy when you consider the great benefits of the north pole. Living things, as well as the human body, function in cycles. To use natural magnetism, you must cooperate with the weekly cycle. If you don't, it will only work for a short while. The wearing schedule is very simple. Wear or use the magnets six days and rest the seventh. A popular strategy is wearing magnetic beads around your neck.

Assistance from the Body with the South Pole

I just said we never use south pole energies for therapeutic reasons, and now I'm going to contradict myself. I call this the old injury strategy. Using this strategy deliberately causes stress and maybe pain to the body. It is used after you lose patience with the strategies mentioned above. Let's say you have a sore neck from a car accident ten years ago. The pain bothers you every day. You place an all-north magnetic wrap directly over the injury. Nothing happens and you are too impatient to continue. You want relief now. The way to get it is to create stress at the site by way of south pole energies.

Turn your uni-pole magnet over and use the wrong side, but no longer than twenty minutes. Then use the north pole. Be prepared to use the magnet for at least three days before you give up. When you use the south pole, you are energizing and further injuring yourself. This signals the brain to send in the troops. The brain takes energy it is using for other things and directs it to this emergency you created. Between the body and the north pole of the magnet, the injury will heal. The pain will go away. I have explained this in terms of a person being impatient. Being in pain is not fun. This method is very successful but should be used with care.

Drink Magnetized Water

This water is sometimes referred to as charged water or electro-changed water. It doesn't matter what you call it as long as it is magnetized with north pole energy. I have noticed that some food supplement companies that sell liquid supplements are "charging" their liquid supplements. Because there is so much confusion in this very simple technology, we can't be sure these manufacturers are magnetizing the food supplements with north pole energy.

To magnetize water, take filtered or spring water and place it on the north pole of a large penetrating magnet. If you leave it in place overnight, you can be sure the magnetizing is complete. By drinking this water, you give your body a head start on pH balancing.

This frees up energy to do other things. It also assists the body in eliminating more poison. Diarrhea is common when people first drink magnetized water. After the initial symptoms of poisons are on their way out, the person feels extra energy. If they have a long-term disease, the body can direct its attention to helping get rid of the disease.

Another thing that has been very successful is to wash your eyes with this magnetized water. The results of this are similar to putting magnets over the eyes. It increases circulation. Magnetized spring water also provides other nutrients the eye may be lacking.

Use Magnets for Energy

Some animals get much of their energy directly from the earth. Examples of such animals are sharks, who get ninety percent, and roaches. For this reason, it is very difficult to get rid of roaches by trying to starve them. Human beings are among these "animals." It is said that humans get about thirty percent of their energy from the earth. Try a simple experiment. Walk barefoot in grass and feel the energy. People were intended to live and work outside, and those who do are healthier than those that do not. Perhaps this is one of the reasons that the game of golf has become popular.

So, let us all quit our jobs, move to the country, grab a hoe, and get busy. Really, we aren't going to do that. In third world cultures, where most of the people do live outdoors, they enjoy very high levels of health. If living outdoors is not an option for you, then the next best thing is to expose your body to magnetic fields as much as possible.

 Energy coming from the north pole of a properly designed therapeutic magnet is the same as the energy coming from the north pole of the earth, that is, if you live in the northern hemisphere. (If you live in the southern hemisphere, you would use the south pole.)

This magnet is a little piece of the earth. Here are some suggestions of ways to increase your energy by using magnets.

☐   **Sleep on a Magnetic Mattress Pad**

When you start sleeping on a magnetic mattress pad, circulation can improve. This means poisons start to leave and sometimes this process can be stressful. The same symptoms of poisoning occur when the poison is coming out as it did when it went in. After the initial poisons leave your body, you will experience more energy than ever before.

These force fields assist the body in healing itself. They can help set pH to the body's ideal level, which averages 7.2. They transfer energy to muscles, soothe nerves, and assist us in falling asleep quickly.

Many times, a magnetic mattress pad solves sleep disorder problems. Many companies make them, but few make them all north pole. Always purchase the best mattress pad you can afford.

☐ **Wear Magnetic Insoles**

The foot is full of acupuncture or acu-pressure points that expel energy into your entire body. North pole energy works with the body for proper energy distribution and healing while south pole energy increases the body's energy in an unnatural way. Wearing insoles that are alternating north and south pole energy back and forth or all south can cause increased pain and even anxiety.

☐ **Sit on Magnetic Cushions**

☐ **Wear All North Magnetic Jewelry, Especially Bracelet**

☐ **Wear Magnetic Hats**

If you want to increase the body's energy, then expose your body to magnetic energy as much and as often as possible.

I am often asked: "Can you overdo it?" The only case where a person can overdo magnetic therapy treatment is when one is bedridden and stays on the magnetic mattress pad all the time. This person should find a way to remove the magnetic pad from the bed for a short amount of time.

Please do not confuse this with being in bed when temporarily sick. When sick, the body needs to restore the proper circulation as quickly as possible, and magnets are the fastest way to restore circulation. Your body needs this healing energy all day long.

Use Magnets for Peak Performance

If you are an athlete, you need every competitive edge you can get. Competition is great. What could you do if you could increase your energy by just 10 percent? Your brain would focus better. Your body would respond better. If you could increase your energy by 20 percent, what could you do?

With energy on a scale from one to 10, with 10 being the most energy your body could ever have, 1 being life sustaining energy, and 0 being dead, you, as an athlete, are probably already functioning in the high end of the scale.

When you approach the high end of any scale, the effort to increase is much greater than in the middle or lower end. For example, it is harder to raise your grade from a "B" to an "A" than from a "C" to a "B." Since an athlete's body is already functioning in the high-energy regions, I cannot really say what the increase will be.

For me, the energy increase was significant. I have always been a visionary with loads of ideas to do things and make them better. I have had hundreds of business ideas. But I had very little energy to make any of my visions a reality. Now that I sleep on a magnetic mattress pad, wear high-powered magnetic insoles, sit on cushions all day, and sometimes wear other magnetic items, I have more energy than I need. I go through an exercise program every morning with ease. I swim and move around the office and house at high speeds. My thinking abilities are better, and I have more energy now than I ever did as a teenager. As a result of all this activity, I have reached my body's ideal weight without paying any attention to losing weight. I regret that I didn't know about magnets all of my life, but I'm glad I found them now.

Chapter Three

The Real World

Anyone can listen to what someone says, but everyone wants to know real-life examples—what really happens. Here are some real-life examples of people just like you and me. Here are things that have happened in the real world.

These Are All Real People with Real Problems Being Helped in A Very Real Way. Magnetic Therapy Works for Everyone.

Cindy, in Rochester, Minnesota, suffered from sinus trouble. She took prescription medicine and got relief from the sinus condition but then suffered from the side effects of the medicine. Her doctor told her the only thing they could do for her was sinus surgery. That was three months ago. She tried medical magnets, and today she is symptom free. She quit taking the medicine and stopped seeing the doctor for sinus trouble.

Mildred, in Elk River, Minnesota, had a car accident over forty years ago. She was a passenger in a car going fifty miles per hour that hit another car head on. She escaped with her life and numerous broken bones, including both legs. Over the years it became harder and harder to walk. Now, in her eighties, it seemed almost impossible to ever be pain free. Doctors could do nothing except re-break the bones and reset them, and it was decided that she was too old, since there were no guarantees that it would help. Every step was painful, and she gained weight due to being inactive. Life, in general, was a great effort. Then, we introduced her to medical magnets. She bought two knee tubes and sleeps in them every night. She has been pain free ever since.

Ed, in Grand Rapids, Michigan, was informed that he suffered from the same severe kind of arthritis that his sister had died from. His hands were blotched from it, and every joint in his body was wracked with pain. When we first spoke to him, he had just taken a prescription painkiller but was still suffering. He decided to try a magnetic bracelet. In less than half an hour, he came back to see us with a big smile on his face. He was opening and closing his hands; his fingers were limber, and his hand was pain free.

Roger, while visiting Quartzsite, Arizona, came by our display at the "Main Event," a famous gem show. We told him about medical magnets. He showed us what he thought was a precancerous sore near his right eye. It was bright red and painful and would not heal. He had, over the last few years, had other skin cancers removed surgically. Roger bought a NeoMax on Friday. He taped it over the sore for thirty minutes in the morning and thirty minutes in the evening for the rest of the weekend and came back to see us on Sunday. The sore was no longer red. The scab was also gone, and it didn't hurt. On Monday, he was so happy he came back again. We could visibly see the sore was getting smaller.

Charley, in Wisconsin, used to suffer from painful knees. When we first met him, he'd had knee surgery and was in great pain. His knee was rubbing bone on bone. He purchased a knee tube, and within two hours the pain was almost gone.

A man in Milwaukee, Wisconsin, bought a magnetic chain for high blood pressure. We spoke to him again a month later. He said his blood pressure hasn't been this close to normal in twenty years. He said that on a scale of one to one hundred, he felt like a ninety-eight.

Jeanne, in Fulton, New York, had a sharp pain in her abdomen that was so severe it caused her to double over in pain. Her doctor said it was appendicitis. Due to a lack of insurance coverage, Jeanne's only alternative was to suffer. Suffer, she did not. She placed the north pole of her medical magnet on the area where there was sharp pain. Within seconds, she could feel it start to subside. She taped it over the painful area for about four hours. The pain never came back.

Donald, in Onalaska, Wisconsin, tapes small gold-plated medical magnets to the magnet points by his ears to restore his hearing. After three months of faithfully taping them in place every morning and every evening for half an hour, nothing seemed to be happening. One afternoon our conversation turned to a dream that Donald had been having. He dreamed he heard chimes just before he woke up. His wife announced, "That's our clock! You aren't dreaming. You are hearing our clock!" Slowly but surely his hearing was coming back.

Linda, from Sedona, Arizona, bought a pair of insoles for herself and her husband. Within minutes of putting them on, she said they made her feel good. After wearing them for a few days, she noticed she no longer got tired in the late afternoon, and she and her husband felt so energized they noticed they were working about three hours longer than before and feeling better.

Steve, from New Jersey, called us about his dad who had been experiencing lower back pain and was scheduled for exploratory surgery. Steve bought our middle of the line mattress pad. The very first night his dad slept on the mattress pad, he experienced more pain than before. The reason this happens is because the force fields penetrate the entire body, and the toxins and poisons that have been lying dormant for many years start dissipating, enter the blood stream, and start moving out through the body's elimination system. This takes about four days. When Steve's dad felt the stress of detoxification, he knew there was something to this and that the medical magnets actually did something. By Wednesday, he was convinced enough to postpone the surgery.

Joanne, in Milwaukee, Wisconsin, had the beginning of carpal tunnel syndrome. Her wrists and hands went numb from time to time. She bought two magnetic wrist wraps and within a few minutes could feel the numbness leave.

Constant wearing of a bracelet on one wrist only will demonstrate the difference. A seventy-one-year old man with arthritis wears one bracelet twenty-four hours a day. The hand with the bracelet is pink with no age spots. The blood vessels are smaller. The other hand is gaunt-looking, and the blood vessels are protruding. It is grayer in color with the wrinkles very pronounced. The hand with the bracelet looks many years younger.

Cheryl, in Richardson, Texas, first tried a magnet to relieve a severe headache. In fifteen minutes, her headache was gone. "I get headaches fairly often, but this magnet always works like a charm," says Cheryl.

A young man who could hardly breathe approached us at a company display last year. His eyes were red and running. I placed two small, gold-plated medical magnets under his nose slightly touching the nostrils, one on each side. I held them there for two minutes. After two minutes, his nose started to run, his eyes were no longer red, and breathing was almost completely restored. A couple more minutes went by and his breathing was completely normal. Three or four hours later he came back to let us know he was still breathing fine and that there was no sign of allergies or any breathing discomfort.

We met a man who had a sore on his foot for two years that he could not heal. He had been in the hospital twice and had taken every antibiotic his doctor tried. The sore was continuously getting worse, and he was facing amputation. I sold him a NeoMax and told him to place it over the sore, taping it there while he slept. Within a week it was almost healed, and two weeks later there was no trace of it.

Debbie told me about her broken finger. She did not go to the doctor because she had experience with broken fingers. She simply went to the pharmacy and bought a finger splint. The pharmacist told her he thought her finger was broken in a number of places. Debbie fastened the splint in place and taped the north pole of a medical magnet over it. Within an hour, the pain was gone. Within three days, she took the splint off, and by the end of the week, the broken bones had healed completely. Debbie told us that she had broken fingers before but never had one heal this fast.

Once when I attended at a pool party in Las Vegas, there were some children playing in the wading pool who were burned by the sun. The children were in a lot of pain. I stroked their painful skin with a NeoMax. A short time later, they said that their pain was gone. They ran back to play in the water. About an hour later, they were back to have me take away the hurt again with my magnet. I saw the children again the next day and was amazed. Their sunburn was not red or blistered, but was tan.

One of our customers had a friend working a show who was in a lot of pain from being on his feet all day. I told this customer that if he would place these insoles in his shoes, he would notice the difference in pain relief within three hours or less. Later in the day, this customer made a special trip back to our booth to let me know I was right. He said that his pain was relieved, but he noticed the pain had started to go away in one hour, not three.

A gentleman came by our booth who had a painful knee. He said there was never a time when the knee did not hurt. I invited him to sit down and take the NeoMax-Gold and place it on the knee. He held the NeoMax-Gold on his painful knee for approximately five minutes. "Does your knee still hurt?" I asked. "No," he said, "not where the magnet is. It hurts everywhere else."

I received a call from a gentleman in Phoenix, Arizona. He had purchased a mattress three weeks prior to his call. He told me that he was in his sixties, and although he didn't want to admit it, his strength was weakening. He realized this a few weeks prior when his wife asked him to open a jar and he couldn't. After sleeping on the magnetic mattress pad for three weeks, he was handed a stubborn jar and opened it with no problem.

He remembered me saying that sleeping on a mattress pad at night can help the body help itself. It doesn't matter what the problem is, the body knows how to heal itself and take care of itself—including strengthen weak muscles.

I received a call from a man who placed the magnetic Skull Cap on his head directly over a wound that was the result of a hair transplant. He was scheduled with six other men who all had the procedure done at the same time. They all went back together for routine checkups and to have the stitches removed. Our man wore the skullcap every evening.

He went back for his first checkup, along with the other men, and the attendant said that his incisions were doing the best. They went back later to have the stitches removed, and his wound area was not red or sore. The other men all had swelling. I had a visit from a neighbor who bought a magnetic bracelet for carpal tunnel syndrome. She was so glad to be out of pain that she came over to let me know that the bracelet worked just like I said it would. The pain went out of her hand and arm in the first few hours of wearing it.

I received a call from a gentleman who bought his wife a High-Powered Headband for her frequent headaches. She took the usual painkillers, but they upset her stomach. We always instruct customers to place the north poles of the medical magnets directly over the painful area.

This usually works, but headaches are complicated. In fact, pain in general can be complicated because the difficulty can be in one place while the pain is in another. This is called referred pain. She tried the headband over her forehead, wearing it like a headband. It didn't work. She wore it backward. It still didn't work. She then tried it around her neck and hasn't had a headache since.

Jerry, in Colorado, had a painful bone spur. To ease the pain, Jerry taped the side of the NeoMax-Gold with the white side down directly over the bone spur faithfully every night. After the first two nights he noticed nothing, but on the third morning the pain seemed to be less. With each morning, the pain seemed to lessen. After about a month, he started to notice the lump was actually smaller. In six weeks, he was pain free; there was hardly anything left of the bone spur.

Diane's daughter had a sore throat for a number of weeks and couldn't shake it. Diane taped the NeoMax-Gold to her daughter's throat and asked her to sleep with it. The next morning when she opened her daughter's mouth, there was no redness in her throat.

Dick, in Alaska, bought a NeoMax-Gold because he was interested in something new. He placed it within easy reach in his kitchen just in case he needed it. He burned himself on a hot pan. He placed the white label of the NeoMax-Gold, which is the north pole, over the burn. In close to thirty seconds, the pain was gone. He put it back in its place. Two or three minutes later the pain came back. He put the NeoMax-Gold on it again. Within a few seconds, the pain was gone again and never came back. The burn quit hurting in seconds and never blistered or peeled.

Sam, a doctor in Cincinnati, works with a woman who has lived eighty percent of her life with severe headaches. He prescribed a Headband and two NeoMax-Golds. If this would have been anyone else, he would have just suggested one NeoMax-Gold, but this woman needed more power—so he thought.

His patient put the Headband on with each NeoMax-Gold positioned at the temples with the north pole down. Her headache was gone within five minutes.

She kept the medical magnets in place for the rest of the day; the next morning she woke up with no headache. During the next day, she thought she was getting a headache, so she put the magnets back on. The headache never returned. The woman has never had a headache since. Her healing was easy, simple, and worked.

Medical Magnets Have Helped with Diseases That Are Without a Real Cure--Such as Heart Disease and Gulf War Syndrome.

A woman named Debbie discovered the importance of medical magnets. Her father was scheduled for open-heart surgery. Debbie noticed how gray her father looked and how terribly short of breath he became with even slow walking. While he was napping, Debbie wrapped her magnetic mattress pad around him.

When he awoke, he looked better; the grayness in his complexion was gone, and he did not seem to get as short of breath when walking from room to room. The day came for his open-heart surgery. Just before the operation a dye test was done to determine exactly where the blockage was. The results came back, and they were perplexed. Something must be wrong with the dye. They did another test. It was the same as the first. The results of the dye test showed no blockage. At all. The operation was canceled.

Magnetic Therapy Works for Professional Athletes, Too.

Marvin Fernandes, a leading wide receiver for the NFL's Los Angeles Raiders, sleeps on a magnetic mattress pad. He testifies, "I don't get tired running. I stay fresh, so I get and stay open. I run right past the younger guys. I go to sleep faster... and it helps keep me at peak performance. It's non-chemical, non-invasive. ..I sleep great. I'm totally rested." Some of his teammates are now using magnetic bed pads.

Tom Hanley used himself as a subject for studying the magnetic mattress pad. He was Mr. Canada, a weight-lifting champion in 1990. He doesn't take drugs, enzymes, or even vitamins.

 He had reached the apex of his career without an increase in the last year and a half. After six weeks of sleeping on the magnetic mattress pad, his exercise program had increased by 46.6 percent.

Muscle soreness was a major problem. After six weeks of sleeping on the pad, soreness was reduced by 80 percent. After the six weeks of sleeping on the pad, his weight dropped seven pounds while his muscle dimensions remained the same.

Bill Romanowski, a linebacker for the Super Bowl champion Denver Broncos, has been using magnets for seven years. "I'm a believer, definitely," he says. "The first time I tried them, I got pain relief."

More Astounding Stories About One of the Leading Killers in The United States Today— Cancer. Yes, Here Are Several Stories of Real People Whose Cancer Has Been Healed.

A bald man had skin cancer all over his head. He placed the north pole side of our gold-plated medical magnets right over each spot of cancer. Within two weeks, every one of the spots were gone. He had gone to the doctor and was told he had melanoma skin cancer and made an appointment to have it removed in two weeks. He obtained some gold-plated medical magnets from us and taped one over each spot on his head. When the day of his surgery arrived, the doctor examined his head and forehead. There was no cancer.

Tricia had a brain tumor. Tricia did not have insurance and didn't have the money to see a doctor. She bought an attractive hat to glue a NeoMax into so the north pole energies would penetrate the tumor continuously. She wore the hat every day and slept in it at night. In just a few days, Tricia said she could feel the tumor move. Within a few weeks, all the symptoms of the tumor were gone, and she made a complete recovery.

Debbie Williams' close friend *Sue* had liver cancer. She had lingered in pain for a number of months and eventually had to enter the hospital. The doctors did everything they could, but her body would not respond to any treatment the established medical community had to offer. The family was notified and many came to the hospital to say good-bye, and the family called the priest to administer Last Rites. The doctor told the immediate family that she would not last through the day and would pass away within a few hours. Debbie took her magnetic mattress pad off her own bed and took it to the hospital and gave it to Sue's daughter. She told her to place it over her mother and to stay with her to make sure it didn't get taken off. The normal way we use the magnetic mattress pads is to lay on them, not put them over us, but in this case, it might become necessary to remove the mattress pad quickly. The little girl peeled the sheets back that covered her comatose mother and placed the mattress pad over her, making sure the north poles were down.

To everyone's surprise, she was alive the next morning. She lived through the rest of that day, as well as Tuesday, Wednesday, and Thursday. On Friday, she woke up hungry! She had completely regained consciousness and seemed to be recovering.

The next Monday, the mother left the hospital and went to a nursing home. Over the next few weeks, she kept the mattress pad around her continuously. At night she slept on it. During the day, she draped it around her as part of her clothing. She felt better and better with each passing day. The family came and took her on outings. She had the joy of seeing and holding her new grandchild.

Unfortunately, the day came when her original doctor called her in for an examination. He was amazed that the tumor had shrunk. He recommended that she go back on chemotherapy. She told him she was alive today because of the medical magnets. He told her the very idea was ridiculous. She obeyed the doctor's orders and put away Debbie's mattress pad.

On September 22, 1995, I got an update on the health of Debbie's best friend, Sue. That day her blood test was 2.5 out of 15 and she was back in the hospital for a blood transfusion. Today she is in and out of consciousness.

When Sue was in the nursing home with the magnetic mattress pad wrapped around her, the doctor examined her, and the tumor was shrinking. Now, she has taken the medical magnets away, and she is again headed for her deathbed.

Chuck Hackney's Story

As a teenager, *Chuck Hackney* took a job as a life guard. One fateful day he dove in the water wrong and hit the bottom of the pool. An ambulance rushed him to the hospital, and he left the hospital on a stretcher paralyzed from the neck down. His future was cut short by one dive into the pool. His parents bought him a magnetic mattress pad and a NeoMax. He sleeps on the mattress pad every night, and his mother rubs his neck with the NeoMax. Since then, she has bought Acupuncture Point medical magnets to place on his body in different places to kill bacteria, heal bed sores, or build weak muscles. Recently, Paulette, Chuck's mother, informed me that they had just returned from a biofeedback session. They placed a probe on a key spot on Chuck's legs and got a response. That means he has the physical ability to walk again.

The following was taken from a letter from *Paulette Hackney*:

"On July 4, 1990, my husband and I were frantically trying to get to Bayfront Medical Center. Our seventeen-year old son, Chuck, had been badly injured in a water accident where he was working as a lifeguard at a popular water park.

They were doing a practice drill when he raced down one of the slides and did not come up. Somehow he had flipped and struck his head on the bottom. He held his breath until rescued by the others and told them he couldn't move."

"Finally, we reached the hospital and were told by his doctor that Chuck had badly bruised his spinal cord at C-34. Chuck would never walk again. Because his injury was so high, he could not breathe on his own for very long. Our world was coming apart. How were we going to tell Chuck about his injury when we knew so little ourselves? Exactly two weeks after the accident, they took him to surgery to fuse C-34. It was at this time they discovered a bedsore about three-inches in diameter and to the bone. This would account for his temperature. Three days after surgery, he developed pneumonia and was no longer able to breathe on his own. For two months he fought for his life. He was put on a respirator and had a tube down his throat and a tube fed. After eighteen days, a tracheotomy was performed.

We watched our son, who was so athletic, drop from 165 pounds to 115 pounds. On September 14th, we were told Chuck was being transferred to the step-down ward. He was skin and bones, but breathing on his own again. That evening we all crowded into his room and on command, he moved his right then his left foot over and over; it was not a spasm, which is common with this kind of injury. Maybe this was a good sign, but it never happened again. On September 17th, he was finally transferred to a rehabilitation center.

By this time, he was in fragile condition. He had bedsores, and they discovered he had a tear in his urethra that would also require surgery. Both surgeries were postponed until he was stronger. At the end of October, he had surgery on his urethra, and one week later surgery on the bedsore. This put him in bed for over a month; it was another month before he was able to sit up.

Because of all the down time, he didn't have much rehabilitation before coming home on January 17, 1991. We were so scared; so much could go wrong. Chuck's nurse, who has been with him since day one, showed us that we could make a difference by working his arm muscles with wrist weights.

He was sure nothing was going to help until one day he moved his left arm just a little. It became clear that if Chuck was to have any chance of getting better, he needed a different doctor. By October of '91, we had an appointment with a medical doctor who specialized in rehabilitation.

Technology and medical research is moving right along, and we want Chuck to benefit from it all. He now rides a computerized bike, with an electric stem hooked into electrodes. He pedals the bike on his own. A small electric stem unit works his arms, lower legs, and feet. Quad pegs help him push his chair. A standing frame takes care of weight bearing.

Through biofeedback, we know he has a lot of activity below his injury. The brain has a greater capacity to learn another pathway. But the muscles must also be strong enough to move the extremity. Chuck works out almost every day. We are willing to try most anything that might help him in some way."

We first met the Hackneys in December of 1994. About a year later, we donated the magnetic equipment mentioned in the "Magnetic Research Protocol" by William H. Philpott.

After he had been sleeping on the magnetic mattress pad for about a year, we visited the Hackney family. Chuck was enjoying a life as active as possible. He bought classic cars and took them to shows to put on display. As soon as he started sleeping on the mattress pad, the bedsores healed and never came back.

From time to time, he would get sores between his toes that became infected. If this happens now, his mother places a powerful magnet directly over the sore; it goes away in a few days. It will be wonderful if Chuck walks again. We have seen many miracles with magnetic therapy, and we believe anything is possible. The following was taken from another letter we received from Paulette, Chuck's mother: "I know people tend to look at alternatives and laugh...I thought magnetic therapy was a joke. Well, because of my son Chuck, I had to know more. I read everything I could get my hands on. The more I read, the more I understood how magnets help the body heal itself, without any side effects. My family and I have seen so many wonderful things happen. Hopefully, the best is yet to come."

When asked how Chuck is doing today, Paulette replied he was doing "good" and is "pushing for better health." When asked if she would remove his magnetic mattress pad, her reply was no she would not. Before Chuck received the mattress pad, he had trouble with his toenails becoming infected. A few days after he would have his toenails trimmed, he would have to go the doctor because infection had set in. Since he has been on his magnetic mattress pad, he has not had this problem. Paulette remarks Chuck's health has been extremely good since using the LGS mattress pad.

Acupuncture Magnets

Early in my "magnetic" career I was selling magnets at a county fair. I went armed with many studies to be able to answer any question anyone could ask. (At least that was my goal.) I had read books on magnetic acupuncture, and this information was fresh in my mind. I recall when a young man, probably in his late teens or early twenties, came by. The ragweeds and pollens were in the air, and this poor man was fighting for every breath. My desire to discover if the magnets would work and my desire to help this young man teamed up.

It is not smart to try something in front of an audience unless you at least have some sort of idea as to what is going to happen. I stepped out on faith. I can scarcely believe what I did.

I asked him if he would like to get help breathing. He said he did. I told him about the magnets and how to use them, showing him that we hold them directly over these points at the lower part of the nose. He asked me how long. I said, "Two minutes." I placed the little magnets at the bottom of his nose and timed the two minutes. When we were about half way through, it was apparent it was working, and I couldn't believe my eyes. His nasal passages were starting to clear up.

We kept the magnets in place the entire two minutes. It was a miracle. His eyes were less red, and he was breathing almost normally. After a few minutes of celebration and small talk, the young man and his friends were ready to leave. He asked me how long the wonderful relief would last. I told him that every person's condition is a little different. I asked him if he would come back in a couple of hours so I could see. He agreed. Three or four hours went by, and he came back. He demonstrated no symptoms of hay fever whatsoever. He was breathing normally; his sinuses were not draining, and his eyes were not watery or red. He told me that after he left, he continued to feel better and better and better.

I could understand the problem clearly since my husband has had breathing problems like this his entire life. When he has problems, I always place the magnets on the acupuncture points at the base of his nose. It worked for him the entire remaining part of the summer and fall.

Then the next summer, about a year later, Lew, my husband, woke up through the night and couldn't breathe. He placed the magnets on the lower part of his nose. He got relief and went back to sleep. He woke up a couple of hours later and couldn't breathe again. He used the magnets with some success but didn't get complete relief as he did in the past.

I was baffled. After a couple of minutes of deep thought, I came up with a theory. If magnetic energy is like a snowplow clearing a highway, then after the highway is plowed, there is no reason to send the snowplow down the highway again. When the highway is clear, it is clear. So why couldn't Lew breathe? He couldn't breathe because there were other highways that needed clearing. So I got the electrical map of the body out and located other points that relate to breathing.

My strategy was hit or miss. I would try one, and if that didn't work within ten minutes, I would try another one. The first one

I selected was on the back. I positioned two magnets directly over these points and taped them in place.

After ten minutes, there was some improvement, but he was still having a difficult time breathing, so I selected another area. All of these points require two magnets—a magnet for each side. This next point was on the wrist.

I decided to use a magnet one inch in diameter and decided to make sure the north pole was inward to the body. This time we had incredible success! Lew could breathe freely within two minutes.

I then told him he could take the magnets off. He did. Right away he started choking up. He put them back, and he could breathe. We figured out a way to secure the magnets in place that would be comfortable for several hours—we used elastic wristbands. Lew wore those magnets for several days. The only time he took them off was to shower.

Probably ten days went by. As long as he wore them, he could breathe. As soon as he took them off, he choked up. Then one day he took them off and left them off. This was such a bad day for hay fever sufferers that the high pollen count was being announced over the radio.

Did Lew have a problem? No. He breathed normally! He didn't need the magnets. It has been five years, and he has not had that kind of allergy type breathing problem since.

Word for Word Excerpts
Lewis Lyon's Radio Broadcast

Caller with Rotator Cuff Injury

Caller: I do a lot of weight lifting you know, and I got myself a pretty good rotator cuff injury.

Lew: Oh really.

Caller: They told me to cut out lifting weights. I've been using that brick on my shoulder for about the last five weeks. I'm still lifting weights. Nobody seems to believe that I'm doing it; and, also, I'm not fully cured; don't get me wrong, I still have an ache, but I take care of that every day. I keep it on there maybe two to three hours during a day. That brick has brought tremendous results.

Lew: That's great!

Caller: This idea that you can't work through a rotator cuff injury—I see a lot of these guys; they got their arms in a sling. I tell them get your arm out of that sling. Get yourself a magnet and you can continue on lifting…..

Lew: Well, some people listen and some people don't.

Caller: I'm really getting good results, and I want to let you know it. As far as that magnetized water is concerned, I've been magnetizing my water for the last month, and, believe it or not, I really feel good.

Lew: That is great.

Caller: Take care, and I'll be talking to you.

Lew: All right. Thanks for calling.

Caller with Knee Pain

Caller: Good evening. I'm the guy with the bad knee. I'm here to tell you that this knee is now absolutely one hundred percent perfect.

Lew: Oh really?

Caller: Yes sir. No aches, no pains, no swelling of any kind. I have, I'd say, 100% strength back in that knee.

Lew: And how long have you had the product?

Caller: Oh, I've had the product now for I don't think quite two months. But the knee actually was almost 100%

better almost two weeks ago. And the more I use it and the more I use the magnetic water, I have absolutely no aches, no kinks, no cramps, no nothing .... I can actually jump up and down on it too. No pain, no discomfort. I mean this knee is absolutely perfect!

Lew: That is just wonderful! You were having quite a bit of trouble with it?

Caller: Oh yes; this knee was swollen to almost twice the normal size when I first came up to your office. I think your wife had seen it. It was quite nasty looking, this knee. Actually, I was thinking about wearing the knee tube on my other knee to get it feeling as good as this knee feels.

Lew: That is tremendous.

Caller: I think I'm going to do that because it's not in bad shape, but you know it could use a little toning up, if you know what I mean.

Lew: Well, it couldn't hurt it, and I would strongly suggest that the bad knee have that knee tube on it every night when you're sleeping for quite some time to give that cartilage a chance tocompletely repair.

Caller: It almost feels like I'm eighteen years old again.

Lew: That's great.

Caller: Once again, I will say to anybody that has any doubts about this—don't be so fast to doubt. I think you would be best off giving it a try. It's well worth your time.

Lew: Yes, sir. I agree. Thanks for calling. I'm sure glad to hear about that knee.

Caller with Foot Problems

Caller: Good evening. I used your insoles for neuropathy of my feet, and it took care of it. I have a question. After the pain stops and it's been OK, do you have to keep using the insoles, or can you leave them off?

Lew: Well, you could leave them off but I'll tell you what. I wear them every day. I don't have anything like that in my feet but I don't want anything there either. And there's 200 acupuncture points in your foot so that magnetic field can help a lot of things in your body besides just your feet.

Caller: Well, I had a problem with one of my feet. I've been wearing them all day and night. That's why I didn't know what to do.

Lew: Well, I wear mine all day. I don't wear them at night.

Caller: I'll try it and see. Thank you.

Lew: You bet.

Bob from Long Island

Bob: I have a good report here. I had a fellow call me that had gotten my catalogue. He has a shop business. His name is John, and he has some bone spurs on his heels and called me up and said he couldn't afford to get operated on because it would take too much time out of his job, because he runs the shop by himself. He went for whirlpool treatments and chiropractor and nothing was helping him.

Then he heard about the magnets. He got my catalogue somehow; and I went over there, and I took two high powered ankle wraps and the foam insoles; and when I came over, he was holding onto the car and limping to come to me, and he had a real depressed look on his face. I said, "Can I try putting them on now. You look like you're really hurting?" So he said, "yes." So I did.

It was the fastest I'd ever seen anything work. I

thought it worked fast on me. But I put the one ankle wrap on while I was getting the other one ready to put on he says, "You know, the pain is going away in my foot," and I didn't get the insoles in his shoes yet, and I tell you when I left there this guy was so happy he was almost crying. He shook my hand. He couldn't believe it.

Lew: That is really great, Bob.

Bob: I never seen anything work that fast. In five minutes, this guy was doing a jig.

Lew: That is really terrific.

Bob: I just wanted to let everybody know this is the second time I've seen this with bone spurs on the heels. It worked really fast. Almost instantly.

Lew: Well, most bone spurs didn't go away for 7-10 weeks, but they dissolve, and they're gone. That's it.

Bob: Yeah, I had told him that. I said to wear it night and day for a week. Just to keep that active there, and he said he would do that. He was just so happy it was unbelievable.

Lew: That is really wonderful. I've seen that many times with people. Thank you for calling.

Jody in Illinois

Jody: I called about a month ago, and I got some of your insoles because I had heel spurs. Well, about a week after using the insoles, I had some slivers up the ankle section by the front of the foot.

After about a week, they felt like they wanted to come out of there. My mother took a knife and cut the spots right out of there. Left two craters in them, but they came right out. I couldn't believe it.

Lew: I can't either.

Jody: Felt like my feet were getting warm, and they were in a sauna. They certainly feel a lot better. I had like dry cracked skin on my feet, and its getting much better.

Lew: That's great. Thank you for calling.

Wrist Wraps

Charlie: I would like to tell you about the wrist wraps you sent me for a young lady that works with me. About a month ago, she came to and said, "My left arm hurts so bad I couldn't even make the bed this morning." So, I called Becky, and she brought her wrist wrap up for this young lady, who works with me. So she started wearing Becky's wrist wrap. Well, last Thursday, a week ago, the order came in for her. She ordered two of the wrist wraps. I took them to work for her on Monday. She wore them all this week.

Lew: How are her wrists doing?

Charlie: She is doing fantastic! Her arms aren't hurting her a bit. Within half a day after putting Becky's wrap on, it started to ease up.

Magnetic Mattress Pad

Caller: I want to share my experiences with the magnetic therapy. Like to say that before we got the mattress pad that morning I went for a walk, and I had a real difficult time trying to walk the half hour that I did. I just did not have the energy. I just couldn't get myself going; and that afternoon we got the mattress pad, and one night on that mattress pad, and the next morning I got up and took a walk again; and I walked for an hour; and I had energy like you wouldn't believe. I was absolutely amazed at that. I had such a wonderful night's rest. It was just amazing to me.

Lew: Well, that's great. I love to hear this.

Caller: I also wanted to say that in sleeping on the mattress pad, I had trouble with a hemorrhoid, and I had been taking herbs. That was the only thing I could find that would keep it in control until I started sleeping on the mattress pad; and it's completely gone. I don't have to take any of the herbs any more, which is wonderful because I'm not a pill person. And I also used the brick on my uterus. I had a fibroid in my uterus, and it took it away completely. The heaviness is gone, the heavy bleeding, the pain.

Lew: I remember you calling me and asking me about that.

Caller: Yes, and I will not have to have surgery, which is wonderful. They wanted to do a hysterectomy. And also, I have the car seat, and it's just been wonderful for my degenerated disc in my back, especially with traveling. I find it just wonderful. So, I really am sold on magnetic therapy.

Lew: Yes, ma'am, I guess you are, and you have a good reason to be. That is really tremendous, and I sure thank you for calling.

Tony from Chicago

Tony: I had to heal my arm. I had a brick, and I had a real bad infection from a cat bite. And I used it then. I kind of stopped using it because, you know, nobody else uses it, so why should I, but I got another infection. I have a habit of biting my nails, and I peeled it down too far, and my finger started to get inflamed. Before I went to the doctor, I put it on the brick for a little while. It took a couple of days because I fell asleep. I couldn't keep it on the brick for more than 10 minutes. After a couple of days, all the inflammation went down and then it healed on its own.

Lew: Hey, that's great, Tony. Let me ask you something. Have you been drinking magnetic water?

Tony: Yes. I have a canteen, one quart, and I put that on the brick overnight; then I put it in the freezer, and I put another canteen on the brick, and I take the frozen magnetic water to work with me. Sort of melts over the eight hours, and I have magnetic water all day. And I have three bricks so...

Lew: I think you have enough bricks to cover yourself.

Tony: One of my cats has allergies, and he was getting injections from the Vet, hydrocortisone, which I don't think is very good for him. I decided to stop going. I just keep the brick under the water dish, and when he puts his face over it to drink, he gets the north pole energies in his face, plus he's drinking the magnetic water; and it seems to keep his eye leakage to a minimum.

Lew: Yes. If you want to do some real good for that cat take an eyedropper and wash that eye out with the magnetic water.

Tony: I heard that's soothing for the eyes.

Lew: You bet. It can really be good for them and might move that infection.

Tony: I forgot about that. I'll have to try that.

Lew: Yes. I've been doing it, and I'll tell you what--it sure makes my eyes feel good.

Tony: Yeah. I tried that a couple times. I should use that on my eyes, too.

Lew: All right, Tony. Thanks for calling.

Magnetic Insoles

Caller: I'm calling in regard to the person that said this thing is hocus-pocus. I can certainly relate to that. He didn't know about the magnetic therapy nor did I. About a month ago, I called your number. You sent me your catalogue. Took about a week. I got the orthopedic insoles for heel spurs, after I had gone through a pair of forty-five dollar insoles from a foot surgeon and that wasn't good enough, so I had to invest another one hundred and ten dollars for a pair of custom made molded type leather insoles. Fine for a while, then I got you. Heard it on the program and ordered the magnetic orthopedic insoles with the exposed magnets and within two weeks time, I've got a pair of new feet, and I want to thank you.

Lew: Well, I'll tell you what. That is just great. Thank you for calling.

Lorraine from Alma

Lorraine: Several weeks ago I called you about a brick.

Lew: Yes. I remember.

Lorraine: I have to tell you I feel so great now--I can't believe it. I put back on 15 pounds.

Lew: Is that right?

Lorraine: Yes. I needed it because I had lost twenty-five pounds and couldn't afford to lose it.

Lew: Is that right, Lorraine?

Lorraine: Yes. I lost twenty-five pounds and looked like skin and bones. I put pants on I hadn't worn for twelve years. Anyway, I used that brick all over. I started off on the stomach. I moved it to the chest cause an x-ray said I had a spot on the chest. I'm not allergic to milk anymore. It worked so well that I ordered the Lone-Ranger Mask. There's something happening with my eyes, but at this particular time I can't tell you what it is. I just know. First, I have to tell you I

have retinitis pigmentosa, glaucoma, cataract
surgery, macular degeneration, so I've got a problem.

Lew: You sure do. I'd say, several problems.

Lorraine: Well, I made one trip to hell. I can't afford another
one. Anyway, whatever is happening, things are
beginning to kind of clear up, it seems like. I have
better peripheral vision, but I've only been using it
three to four weeks. So as soon as it goes a little
further, I'll call you back and tell you. But the brick
is just fine. I couldn't afford the mattress, but the
brick--I put the brick all over. Put it on the arteries.
I believe they call them the carotid arteries. Put it on
my head for an hour. Works very well, and I can't
understand why anybody would be afraid of it. I've
never felt so good in my life.

Lew: That is just wonderful, Lorraine, and I really
appreciate the call.

Caller with a Knee Injury

Caller: I was up at Holmen about two weeks ago. Came in
and bought the brick, the NeoMax and the Knee
Tube. I talked to you ever so briefly when you called
the office.

Lew: I remember that.

Caller: OK. Well, I'll tell you what my experiences are. Now,
as I explained to your wife, I had a knee injury, and
my knee swelled up very bad. The doctor had to take
three vials of fluid out of there. Well, there was still
some swelling, but since I've used the knee brace in
conjunction with the NeoMax and at night sleeping
with the brick under the crook of the leg, I can feel
the knee getting stronger. So I'm saying I am very
pleased with these products.

Lew: Well, I'm glad to hear that, and thank you for calling and telling us.

Caller: Plus, I've also been doing the magnetic water, and I heard your statement about how it can help clear your entire system out. And I will say this: yes, it does! I found it very effective and, in general, I feel much better by drinking it.

Lew: That is great.

Don from Canada

Don: A neighbor of ours came over the other night and he was all busted up with a cold pretty good. So I took my wristband off and put it on him; and the next day it was totally broke up.

Lew: Where did you put it on him?

Don: On his right wrist.

Lew: Is that right? Just on his wrist.

Don: That's all I had available. I wasn't gonna give him my brick. I wear the magnetic insoles, and I use the brick; and I put in on my chest, and I've been up in Oakville and you know how all the pollution stuff is up in there. And I came back with no colds. No, nothing.

Lew: Yes, Don. I've been sleeping on a magnetic mattress pad for almost seven years now, and I haven't had a cold or the flu in seven years; I don't catch them anymore.

Don: Well, this is the same thing with me now. I had a thing out of my head, a one-inch in diameter about three inches thick. I haven't heard any lab reports back, but apparently I was supposed to be in pain. I didn't have any because I'd been listening and using the magnetic water; and when I was up there, unknown to them, I put the brick underneath the water in the day time and they were drinking the magnetic water, too. But anyway, the long and the short is I wash my eyes with magnetic water. I drink it, but I also wash my head with magnetic water every night. And this thing has healed up beautifully.

Lew: Great. It's gone then. Just healing up.

Don: Well, it's pretty ... They can't even find the sucker.

Lew: Great!

Don: I haven't used aspirin in the last eight months from the time I got that thing. No Rolaids; the last time I saw the doctor he sent me for an electrocardiogram because I had something, and he thought it could be a heart attack. And he never did the blood work when he had me there; and that was the first time he had me there in twenty years. So I'll take the magnets over a doctor any day of the week.

Lew: Thank you, Don, and thank you very much for calling.

Magnetic Water

Caller: Yes, sir. I just called to tell you how it helped me.

Lew: Great.

Caller: Well, one thing: the brick brought my blood pressure down.

Lew: It did?

Caller: Another thing. It seemed like sometimes with my heart I could feel a thump in it like a missed beat. Well, it took that out.

Lew: It did?

Caller: Yes, sir. Like a ton of weight lifted off my chest even though it weighs five pounds. Magnetic water. My wife was a skeptic, and she was skeptical from the start. But I listened to you a long time, and I am convinced. Now she is convinced because this magnetic water has got her bowel movements regular. She feels better. She isn't crabby any more; and she had a sore breast. Got your five by seven heavy duty ones, and the pain is gone out of one of her breasts. Didn't come back. People out there: get them while you can. Thank you, sir.

Lew: Thank you very much for calling back.

Magnetic Brick

Ed: I want to relate something about that brick. You know, that brick has been magic for me. About a week ago I tried to get up and my eye was watering real bad and ached in my right and I thought, "Oh, God! Do I have to go to an eye doctor?" So I thought, I'm going to try that brick. I put it on there for about 45 minutes on, 45 minutes off. By the time I went to bed that night, bingo! All gone.

Lew: Great. Wonderful!

Ed: I'll tell you, that brick is the most versatile thing I have ever had.

Lew: Yes, it is.

Ed: I just wanted to relate to you what it can do.

Lew: Thank you very much, Ed. Take care of yourself.

Dalmatian with Food Poisoning

Caller: I have a full-blooded Dalmatian dog, and about two months ago she got food poisoning; and she swelled up around her abdomen and her liver stopped functioning, and she looked like she was pregnant and ready to have twenty puppies. When I took her to the veterinarian, she was developing a heart murmur, and I asked the Vet what I could do. He said everything was hopeless. Just let nature take its course.

Lew: Oh, really.

Caller: I put the dog on nothing but magnetic water, 3,500 milligrams of garlic oil capsules, double dose of dog vitamins, put her on good dog food; and between all that...in a week and a half you should see her. All the bloat went away, and she's her slim, trim self. She's totally healthy. She's just tickled to death.

Lew: That's wonderful.

Caller: And, I give most of the credit to the magnetic water. Because I figured it probably was between that and the garlic. It probably flushed a lot of whatever the poisons were that were stuck in her system.

Lew: You bet it did. It surely did.

Caller: And you know what else I did? I called the Vet back, and I made sure and told him exactly what I used; and he said he's still skeptical, but at least this time when he comes along with another hopeless situation, hopefully he'll suggest it.

Lew: Well, I hope so, but I have my doubts.

Caller: OK, thank you.

Lew: Thanks very much for calling, and I'm sure glad your dog is better.

Caller from Texas

Caller: I wanted to pass the word on down here in this southern climate about fire ant bites. They work beautiful. The quicker they get on the bad set of bites, the better they are.

Lew: For putting the magnetics on the bite?

Caller: Right.

Lew: And it takes that sting and all that stuff right out of them, doesn't it?

Caller: Yes. It does a beautiful job.

Lew: Yes, I know a bee sting is the same thing. I got stung by a bee not long ago and I put a magnet on it and the pain was gone in a matter of seconds.

Caller: Yes. I've had that happen, too.

Lew: And it didn't even swell.

Caller: Yes. We've had that happen. Wife had it happen to her. I put it on there. Within thirty seconds just never did anything, but the fire ants down here is...we don't get stung by bees too much in Texas, but we sure get fire ant bites.

Lew: You get them in Florida, too. I know because I got into a nest of them one-day.

Caller: You're out there working in the garden, and they'll get you.

Lew: Alright, sir. Thanks for calling.

Mary from Ohio

Mary: I'm the one that called about our little grandson with the seizures.

Lew: Yes.

Mary: Well, he's doing great. But I have a question for myself.

Lew: Mary, how great is he doing?

Mary: He has gone from five hundred seizures a day down to two.

Lew: He actually had that many in a day?

Mary: Yes. The tests at children's hospital said he had five hundred a day.

Lew: Wow.

Mary: So, he is doing great. And, I want to tell you I went with my daughter to the neurologist last week and she mentioned the magnets and it just kind of went over his head. As I said, I have a question for myself. I've had open-heart surgery; had a mechanical valve put in, and I've been on Cumadin for five years, and they say I will be on it for the rest of my life. Is there an alternative?

Lew: Well, you should be on the high-powered mattress pad and you should be using the brick on that heart as much as you can.

Mary: OK.

Lew: And very possibly it'll correct that situation, yes.

Mary: What about magnetized water?

Lew: That should also be a great help to you.

Mary: Really.

Lew: Yes. Because it can flush out all the toxins in your body's system. It can get any parasites or anything like that in there—regulate your bowel movements really good; clean out your kidneys, your liver--everything in your system--even your lymphatic system, and with the increased circulation you should feel much better.

Mary: Well, I have circulation problems and so you say the magnetic mattress and the brick.

Lew: Yes.

Mary: Now, would that mean I would get off the Cumadin?

Lew: Many people have. You're going to find out you'll know because your body is your best teacher. That is almost everybody that I've ever put on magnetic therapy that's been on any kind of these petrochemicals has found that when they start with magnetic therapy they become extremely more effective. And you have to cut back as your body tells you you're getting too much. Then you start cutting back—cutting back and, just like Ben, he's clear off his insulin and everything now.

Mary: Right. Well, I'll just have to give it a try. Thank you so very much.

Lew: I'm delighted that you called, and give that little boy a hug for me.

Mary: I sure will.

Lew: That's the best story I've heard in five years.

Mary: Well, great. And I know that we're really pleased.

Lew: That's wonderful. I'm so delighted for you.

Mary: I'm glad that we heard of you and the magnetic therapy.

Lew: OK. Thanks a lot.

Asthma

Caller: I just purchased a magnetic belt, and I have to say that I had it for four days. I have arthritis in my last three vertebrae, and the first two days I wore it all day long and I actually slept with it. I'm a construction worker. I cannot believe the difference in my lower back. I've tried everything: herbs, chiropractor. It's amazing. I don't know how it works. I really don't care. I just know it works, but I do have one question. I heard you talking about it helping asthma.

Lew: Yes sir.

Caller: Now, I have a golden retriever who is ten years old. She has asthma.

Lew: A dog. A dog has asthma? That's the first time I've heard of that.

Caller: Well, I think my vet said that. He was born in Arizona. We moved to Ohio and just recently within the last half-year, when he goes outside, and comes back in during the wintertime, it's that wheezing and heavy coughing sound. So…

Lew: And the vet says its asthma.

Caller: Well, what would you think it is?

Lew: I have no idea. I've been suffering with asthma since I was nine, so I know a little about what magnetic therapy will do for it from first hand experience.

Caller: The thing is I have this belt and I'm saving up to get the brick, but can I use the belt to magnetize the water?

Lew: Sure.

Caller: How long would it take?

Lew: Which belt do you have? Gold or silver?

Caller: The gold.

Lew: Gold belt.

Caller: The brand new one. Kind of goes out towards the tailbone type.

Lew: Take your belt, put a half-gallon jug of water on top of it and lay it on its side so you're touching as many of the magnets as you can. And you probably leave it on there a couple or three hours and it'll be magnetized.

Caller: Oh, great. Great. Yes. Because she wanted to give him all kinds of pills and everything and I heard about this and I then figured, well, I'm going to save up for the brick, and then I was wearing this, thought well, wait a minute. Maybe I can do the same with this belt until I get the money saved for the brick.

Lew: Right. Another thing you can do is take that belt, fasten around that dog's chest area where his lungs are—bronchial tubes—I suppose he has them just like we do.

Caller: Yes.

Lew: And watch in ten minutes if that doesn't subside.

Caller: I'll be dog gone. Yeah. Because I took him in for x-rays and I'll tell you because I was real concerned about it and the x-rays came back and she says he's got a good heart and everything. I don't think it's that.

Lew: What exactly do you feed him every day?

Caller: When he gets his food, he gets a little parsley, a clove of garlic. Garlic is good for humans. I figured it is good for the dog, too. But I want to thank you for the information because I was channel surfing on the shortwave and I heard about the magnetic treatment, and hey, if there's anybody out there who has any doubts…hey, I'm a believer.

Lew: Well, I certainly appreciate your call, sir, and I'm sure there's a lot of people out there who are appreciating it, too.

Caller: Well, I want to thank you, and God bless you and your family.

Lew: Thank you very much.

Magnetics with an Artificial Joint

Caller: I would like to reveal a story that might help your listeners. I have a friend that's a beautician. She fell down and slipped in a beauty shop; a bone came out of her arm, and she had to have an artificial joint in her arm, but she used magnets and lineaments. The doctor told her she'd never be able to use it again and she's right back at work working 10 hours a day.

Lew: Thanks for calling.

Poison Ivy

Caller: I'd like to report on a recovery from poison ivy. I took a NeoMax and left it on overnight. There was pretty much nothing there in the morning.

Lew: Where was it on you?

Caller: It was on my left hand, top of my left hand, sir, and it shrunk it up like it had gone through a process of a week, but it only took overnight.

Lew: I'll be darned. Isn't that great?

Caller: Yes, sir. 'Cause I'm highly allergic to it. I get it a lot.

Lew: Well, just keep that NeoMax in your field pack or your pocket when you're out in the woods.

Caller: Well, sir. We just wanted to let your people, everyone, know it really did take it away. It really worked.

Lew: Well, thank you very much for calling.

Magnetic Brick

Caller: I ordered the brick. I have a son that came down with this disease "physcodosis." He has a lot of pain from arthritis in his knees, elbows, and everything. Because I've been listening to your program a long time and he's just 34 years old and sometimes you can't even get him out of bed. I took the brick in there and I laid it down behind his knee. Five minutes later he called me and said he didn't believe it. He said, "Dad, the pain is gone." I took the brick and put it under the other leg. Ten minutes later he was up walking around.

Lew: Isn't that wonderful?

Caller: And just today—I suffer with congestion—I was coming home with my wife in the car and I could feel—we were going down this bumpy road—I could feel the water fluid shaking around my heart. I got home, got in bed, and laid down on that brick. About 15 minutes later all that was gone. And I just want to thank you for putting this product out because I know what it did for me and my son and a other people.

Lew: Yes, sir. It sure has.

Darrell from Toronto

Darrell: Just wanted to comment. I received the knee tube and I had pain in my left knee for many years after a foolish accident when I was younger, but the pain has now subsided, if not completely gone after wearing it in the evening when I'm sleeping. But, there is a cyst that I believe has developed because of the injury just above that knee. Would a stronger magnet be needed or necessary to dissolve it?

Lew: Yes. And I tell you what I would do. How big is it?

Darrell: Smaller—much smaller than a pea--maybe like two grains of rice. That size.

Lew: OK. You could use one of our dominoes and slide it inside the knee tube right over that sore and wear that every night while sleeping and that cyst can heal.

Darrell: So, the domino could be used for other ailments as well?

Lew: Oh, yes. People have used them for headaches and all kinds of things.

Darrell: Well, where would they place them for headaches?

Lew: On your temple. With a headache you kind of have to feel around your head with a magnet to figure out where it's coming from. But, generally, right in the middle of the forehead is a good place or on either temple.

Darrell: 'Cause that's something I wanted to—actually the knee tube is the first item that I've purchased and I've had good success with it so most likely I'll be getting the domino.

High Blood Pressure

Caller: My wife got that Himalayan type of necklace and it seems to be working pretty good on her blood pressure.

Lew: It's dropped down quite a bit?

Caller: Yes. Its mainly been staying down pretty good. She gets too low then goes too high, so I think its going to level out.

Lew: That's what it's supposed to do and what it's done for many people.

Caller: Thank you sir.

Lew: Thank you for calling.

Leg Amputation

Caller: I would like to pass on a thing that's happened with a friend of mine. He is 89 years old and has very, very poor circulation in his legs. Actually, two years ago they were going to amputate. But he had a heart attack before, so they decided they wouldn't and he's just been struggling along now to the point he can hardly walk with the cane, just getting around a little bit. He saw two specialists. They said there's nothing more they can do for him. Now, I gave him a pair of magnetic insoles. Within days his pain was gone from both legs. He's not using his cane. He went to the mall with his wife, which was the first time in months, and months, and months. He went back to his doctor last week and walked in there without a cane, and the doctor was totally blown away.

Lew: I'll bet he was.

Caller: You, know, I thought it was really wonderful. Now the one thing I must mention: it is a different make and it's the alternating.

Lew: Now, I would strongly suggest he gets on north pole only. Because if he gets any infection he's going to have a terrible time with that south pole energy.

Caller: Yes. Of course he takes them off at night. I knew this when I gave them to him, but I thought, well, if it helps the circulation, which it definitely has, but I thought it was really amazing.

Lew: North-pole energy only will help the circulation more, because south pole restricts circulation.

Caller: Well, it's doing something. It really did a marvelous thing for the circulation.

Lew: He could probably use a pair of high-powered insoles or even the foam insoles, but I would strongly suggest he gets off that south pole because many times these symptoms return with south-pole energy, and then they get worse. Forty years of research by two guys named Davis and Rawls have proven that.

Caller: Is that right?

Lew: Thank you for calling.

Pat from Long Island

Pat: I just wanted to give you an update. I was diagnosed with breast cancer nine months ago. I used the brick, I slept on the mattress pad, drank the magnetic water. I aided the magnets with a change of diet, like Dr. Philpott talks about in his Oxygen/Cancer Book. And so that was almost ten months ago, and I didn't have surgery or chemotherapy or radiation, and I just had another checkup. I had my blood work done to have my tumor marker done and to keep track of my blood because when you have cancer, your blood is really low in just about everything. So, all that has improved and my cancer marker was completely clear again, and my doctor just thinks its an absolute impossibility.

Lew: He does.

Pat: Yea. He's really starting to scratch his head.

Lew: Well, young lady, I sure appreciate the call.

Pat: Well, you're most welcome.

Sue from Maine

Sue: I called about two weeks ago and ordered a skullcap.
          I have Parkinson's disease.

Lew: Yes, ma'am.

Sue: Just got the cap yesterday, so haven't had it long
          enough to give it a real fair trial, but I noticed results
          almost immediately. Yesterday I walked down to the
          community room and when I was done visiting down
          there I got up out of the chair and walked clear back
          to my apartment without holding on to anything. For
          me this is extremely unusual. I have to lurch and
          hang onto things as I go.

Lew: Praise the Lord. I'm telling you, from what I've seen
          of results with Parkinson's, you keep that skullcap
          on as much as you can.

Sue: Well, I have it on as I'm speaking. I feel I have a
          future. I'll keep working on it. I have faith. I know it
          will.

Lew: You keep me advised, won't you? Thanks for calling.

Nell from North Carolina

Nell: I have arthritis in my hip, and I could hardly walk
          because when I get up in the morning I'd have to hold
          on to get around. I'm a very skeptical person. I don't
          believe half of what I hear and half of what I see.
          But anyway, I said something had to happen. I had
          been to the doctors. I have spent thousands of
          dollars on arthritis medicine. It gave me an ulcer, and
          then I lost the feeling in my feet and legs, the nerves.

I could hardly walk. My feet hurt me so bad that I could hardly hobble across the floor.

Well, anyway, after listening to your program, my husband suggested, let's try it. I said, "Well, I don't know. I spent three thousand dollars last year. It won't hurt to spend a little bit more. So I ordered a pair of insoles, mattress pad, the seat cushion, the NeoMax, the dominoes, the Lone Ranger Mask, and the Brick.

Lew: Well that's a good start, ha, ha.

Nell: I only got the products Monday. Already, my feet don't hurt; my legs don't hurt. I feel a little tingling still in my feet because of very little circulation.

Lew: Yes. It's restoring your circulation down there. That's why.

Nell: I had no circulation, and I'm telling all these people out there that might be skeptical. I know. I was. I've been fooled before but this is true. This works. If I say that it works, it works. Lew, I would not ever go back to the doctor. He gave me some pills for circulation in my legs that actually, when I read up on it--it said it was for people with seizures and the side affects of it were hallucinations; it made me dizzy. When I'd get up, sometimes I'd stagger around. I just had to quit taking it but it did help some in my feet and legs, but I couldn't take it for the side affects.

Lew: That's true of many of the pharmaceuticals.

Nell: And I'm telling you people out there listening: This works. If it made my feet and legs—I thought my stuff would come last Friday, but it didn't get here till Monday and I sit on that back porch looking for the UPS man, praying it would come, 'cause nothing else was working. I was in such agony. I had to lay in bed half of the time. Now I can get up and walk. I can do my work. I'm still not completely—I have a little pain in my hip but nothing like it was.

Lew: Well, we can't build Rome in a day, you know.

Nell: No. I probably won't get over it in a day, but it's ninety percent better.

Lew: That's wonderful. That is just wonderful.

Back Injuries

Caller: I injured my back about two and one-half years ago. I was a truck driver and never had a problem with my back for all the years I drove. Then I bent over and tried to pick up a 90-pound tarp and blew out discs and everything else.

Well, they went through therapy with me for about six months. It didn't do any good. Then they operated on it. That seemed to work for about 30 days, then came back worse than ever. Had more therapy and still didn't do any good and basically the doctor said my back was 30 years older then I am. I am 53 years old.

Lew: Oh, so you got an 83-year old back, huh?

Caller: Yes. I asked him if he could get me a new transplant, but he said, "Nope." The pain was excruciating at night. If I could get two hours sleep that would be good, then just up with the pain. Daytime most days I'd just hobble around or sit in a chair and it would be excruciating.

About four months ago, I got one of your Gold series mattress pads, and I'll admit I was quite skeptical about it, but I was to the point that I'd try anything. The first night I had it, I slept the night through for the first time in two and one-half years. It was the first morning I could stand up and not have it take 15 minutes to unfold into a vertical position. The speed is absolutely amazing, and this was to a skeptic myself. This is real relief from long-lasting chronic pain.

Lew: Boy, I'm sure happy to hear that, I'll tell you.

Caller: For your listeners that are listening, I would say that at night my pain relief was in the 80% range, which is just a Godsend. I praise the Heavenly Father for that and the people who supplied this therapy. Compared to what the doctors offered, which was absolutely nothing for their high-priced operations, your pads work. I've been on it about four months, and I plan to stay on it.

Lew: Thanks for the call; take care and keep me posted.

Caller: You too, Lew. I'll be calling you back sometime in the future.

Webb from Michigan

Webb: Just thought I'd call you and tell you--my wife, a couple months ago, bought the beauty mask and since that time she hasn't had to take any allergy pills or anything. She'll wear it in the morning for about an hour and in the evening again. And, she hasn't had to take the pill since she started wearing it.

Lew: Is that right?

Webb: It took care of the sinuses. This is what used to bother her eyes. They would swell up. That beauty mask does more than just beauty.

Lew: Yes. That is an amazing piece of equipment because it can do a lot of things.

Webb: I split my thumb. A board kicked back on me on the saw. I let it bleed to clean it out a little bit, then I put that magnet on there and it stopped bleeding in just a few seconds. Those magnets took the pain out of that, too. It's amazing what it does.

Lew: Yes. It is. I certainly thank you for calling.

Magnetic Brick

Caller: About a week ago, I was walking around the house barefoot and I bumped my big toe. I not only bumped it--I got it caught under about an inch space, and I went down, and oh, boy, I did a beautiful job on it. Right away I went downstairs and got the pillow, doubled it up, and put my foot on the brick and the pain subsided about 60-70% within 10-15 minutes and right now it's been about a week. It all turned black and blue, you know. And right now there's hardly any pain in it and the swelling's just about gone down. Normally, when I've done that before, mostly on my little toe, it would be couple-three weeks before it would be normal. So, that brick sure does work wonders for a lot of different things.

Lew: It is very versatile--that is true.

Caller: Keep up the good work, Lew.

Lew: OK. Thanks for calling.

Ruth from Canada

Ruth: I ordered your magnetic insoles because I had spurs on both heels and I just want to let you know that it really does work, and they are gone.

Lew: How long did it take, Ruth?

Ruth: I'd say, about three months.

Lew: Well, that's longer than normal. They must have been pretty big.

Ruth: Yes. They were, and I still wear them in my runners all the time.

Lew: Yes. Well, I wear them every day all the time because

I don't want any problems with my feet.

Ruth: Exactly.

Lew: I have none, but yes, I've seen that happen many times, Ruth, with these heel spurs. All it is, is a calcium build-up.

Ruth: What causes that?

Lew: Well, your body isn't metabolizing that calcium, so it starts building up in different places. That's what is the main cause of arthritis. And just like an old water pipe in many homes that I serviced with magnets 10-11 years ago, I've seen pipes that started out two inches in circumference and they were down to a pencil size where the water could come through because of the lime and calcium build-up in there. We put very high-powered magnets on those water pipes and in 90 days all that stuff was gone. It does the same in the human body.

Ruth: Right.

Lew: If you look in our catalogue, you will see a picture of what the calcium molecule looks like under a microscope and what it looks like after it passes through a magnetic field. It's much easier for your body to metabolize in that state and it can't stick anywhere. Not only that but it picks up all the stuff that's building and takes it out over a period of time, which is exactly what happened in your heels.

Ruth: Yes. Because I had them in both feet.

Lew: It must have been painful walking around.

Ruth: Believe me, it was.

Sinus Problems

Caller: I would like to talk about excessive mucous. Whenever I have a cold, my sinuses are all stuffed up.

I use the brick in a pillow. It's not very comfortable, but in a few hours, or by morning, my nose will completely drain out. Now, this is a problem because it drains onto the brick. But, also, I noticed that if I get only four or five hours sleep and I'm using the brick either under my pillow or on top of it on the north side, I'll feel more like I got eight hours sleep. And during the day, I'll have more energy to work with.

Lew: Yes, sir. Magnetic therapy can increase your energy. You can bet on that. Are you using magnetic water?

Caller: Yes. I do.

Lew: OK. Because that can help that sinus condition measurably.

Caller: Well, I wasn't drinking the water but when I laid my face on that brick, I tell you, it just drained everything out.

Lew: That I've seen many times, not just with the brick but with the sinus mask and even putting two magnets at each side of the nose in the crevice by the nose on the right and left sides and holding them there even for two minutes. I've seen people just drain like crazy.

Caller: Now, this is the sinus mask?

Lew: Yes.

Caller: OK, but one thing I noticed for sure was the energy. I didn't always do that, but if I got to get up early in the morning and I stayed up too late listening to short wave or watching my favorite Kevin Costner movies, I'll just use the brick as a pillow, and I'll feel great the next day.

Lew: That's wonderful, and I congratulate you in finding that out because your energy levels can go right through the ceiling sleeping on a magnetic bed.

Caller: Yes. I'm going to have to get one of those mattresses. All I have right now is the brick, but I'm getting by. I'll have to get the mattress.

Lew: Thanks for calling.

Ed from Arkansas

Ed: In conjunction with magnetic water I've been drinking when I get out of the shower, I've been taking magnetic water and splashing it on my hair, and I noticed immediately when I brush or comb my hair I don't come out with a handful of hair. I can't afford to lose too much up there, and splashing magnetic water on my hair when I get out of the shower has helped tremendously.

Lew: Yes, Ed, and I've had several people call and tell me they were washing their hair with magnetic water, and it's doing wonders for their hair.

Caller: Right. It gives your hair more body.

Lew: Yes.

Caller: OK. Keep up the good work. Talk with you later.

Lew: Thanks for calling.

Back Pad

Caller: What you have sent me works like a charm.

Lew: Great. What kind of problem did you have?

Caller: Well, I was comatose for three one and half months and then started to try to walk again with difficulty and that Back Pad seemed to take the ache and the pain away. I don't think all that time I had a wedge between my legs and that could have maybe caused a little bit of the problem, but now I'm walking without a walker or a cane.

Lew: Well, that is wonderful.

Caller: And I did not know I had a problem with circulation in my hands. It was very difficult to make a complete fist. Therefore, I got your Wrist Wrap, and I think I could probably climb a tree again.

Lew: That is so great.

Caller: Well, I thank you and your company for being able to rehabilitate me in such a short period of time, and I feel just fine, and I thank you all and both from the bottom of my heart.

Lew: Thank you, sir, for calling. I really appreciate it.

Caller from Indiana

Caller: I bought some of your magnets, and I want to give a testimonial. The massaging insoles. The plastic ones. Within 1 ½ - 2 days, sore feet that have afflicted me for a long time ceased to be a problem.

Lew: That is great.

Caller: And I also bought two of your high-powered wrist wraps because I had injured my left wrist back in March, and I have gotten some really wonderful, wonderful, wonderful, good results. I bought one for each wrist. I said I'm not going to fool around with this. I bought two of them, but I did have one experience, which I'd like to warn your readers about. I attended a seminar at work on computer training and those magnets got near the screen and kind of discolored it.

Lew: Oh yeah. That happens once in a while. You must have been pretty close to it with them.

Caller: Well, I didn't realize what I was doing because all of a sudden I'm pulling about the brightest glowing colors you can imagine all over that screen.

Of course, the seminar leader saw what I had done

with the screen and was horrified. Magnets near a computer: NO, NO, NO!

But, anyway, I'm getting great results with your products. I do have one brief question. I was in an automobile accident. The car was not hurt. No other cars were involved, but slick roads turned the car around in the ditch, and I got my upper back and shoulder jammed up. I'm getting chiropractor care and massage therapy for it. Do you have any recommendations of products I could use?

Lew: Where is the injury in the back? What part of the back?

Caller: Upper back.

Lew: Yes. I'd use a gold wrap on that.

Caller: Gold wrap, and for the shoulder pain?

Lew: Shoulder pain. We have a shoulder harness for that.

Caller: Well, I love your products, and I have had wonderful dealings with your company. Your office staff has always been more than helpful, and God bless and continued success.

Lew: Thank you, sir. Thanks for the call.

Ken from Louisiana

Ken: Just wanted to say I purchased a magnetic belt three months ago, and I just want to say I had back surgery and I used the magnets right after surgery. I got on it-used it seven days straight. Left it on daytime and night and it's been two weeks since I had surgery and I'm walking around. I can bend easily, and it's healed really quick.

Lew: That's great, Ken. Thank you very much for the call.

Headaches

Caller: I ordered some products and one of them was the

headband, and since I am plagued with headaches a lot, I just put that headband on and in a short time it clears up. So I thought perhaps some of your other listeners who get headaches might like to know that.

Lew: Well, I certainly appreciate your call because, yes, a lot of people around the country that are listening will. These headbands and skull caps can be used for serious headache problems.

Caller: You know, I'd like to have a lot of your products, but I just can't do it now, but if I ever can, I would like to order some more such as a skullcap—although I don't have serious health problems. But all the products sound so great. I really would order more if I could.

Lew: Are you drinking magnetic water?

Caller: Yes. I use it to magnetize water, and I believe that helps. My stomach feels better when I drink it and it doesn't puff up as much. It doesn't get that puffy feeling.

Lew: Well, that's great. And your energy level. Noticed a change in that?

Caller: Yes. I do seem to have some more energy. I probably don't drink as much water as I should. It's always been difficult for me to drink as much water as I should, but this water seems to go down easier, and I can tell a difference when I'm away from home and I don't have the magnetized water. My stomach will puff, and I feel uncomfortable.

Lew: That's great, and we sure thank you for calling.

Rich from West Virginia

Rich: I'd like to tell you a success story about your magnetic brick. I had a prostate problem that bothered me quite a bit. So, the doctor gave me Proscar, and I used it about six months. Didn't faze it. I got the brick from a friend of mine who is a salesman for you, and it wasn't three days and I have no prostate trouble and haven't had for five months.

Lew: How about that? Three days.

Rich: It stopped it--just like you turn a light off.

Lew: Isn't that great?

Rich: It's fabulous, and a prostate problem is probably the most miserable problem a man can have.

Lew: Tell me about it. I went through the same thing.

Rich: Right, and I used that Proscar for a long time and that medication didn't do nothing and my brother told me about this brick that helped him so I got one of them and that's money very well spent.

Lew: Well, thank you for calling, Rich, and I'll tell you what- It got rid of my problem, too, only it took me a lot longer than three days.

Rich: Is that right?

Lew: Yes. But I had a serious problem because mine got to the point where it swelled up to where it cut off the bladder. Then, the kidneys stopped, and I was in serious shape for about three days. Finally, found out how to drain, got that drained out and started using magnets on it, and it's taken, oh, I guess, three or four months, and everything is back to normal.

Rich: Well, mine is completely back to normal. Within three days, I could really see a difference.

Lew: Well, you got to it early enough to do that, I guess.

Rich: I'm on the road quite a bit, and I just leave it in my truck. I just sit on it when I'm driving my truck, and that's all I used it and it took care of it. I advise, if anyone's got that problem, get that brick.

Lew: OK. Thank you very much.

Nancy from North Carolina

Nancy: I'm just calling to tell you we received one of your bricks, and I'm a mother of three children. I have ten-month-old twins.

Lew: Oh, how wonderful!

Nancy: Thank you. When I received your brick, my children were very sick at the time with a severe cold. One of the twins was born with pneumonia in the lungs, and we were afraid we might have to take him back to the hospital to get fluid cleared out of his lungs. As soon as we got that brick, we put it on his back. It has cleared that fluid right out of his lungs, and he's doing a lot better.

Lew: How about that? That is really wonderful.

Nancy: Well, I wanted to tell you that brick has been wonderful! The magnetic therapy has been good. One of my children suffers from constipation. I put magnetized water in their formula, and it has cleared right up.

Lew: I found that out real quick the first couple of days I started drinking 6-8 glasses a day. I found out it's impossible to be constipated.

Nancy: Right. We also have realized that since we've gotten the brick. We should have gotten two actually, because we're always fighting over the brick and who's going to get it. But I just wanted to call and let you know it has been wonderful for my family and my babies especially.

Lew: Well, I'm certainly glad you called. I really, really love to hear this, and you give those two little babies a great big hug for Lew, will you?

Nancy: OK. I sure will. Thank you so much.

Lew: Thanks for calling.

Foot Pain

Caller: I bought a Brick and a NeoMax-Gold. I had severe pain in my feet. Well, the pain is gone. It works. I'm drinking the magnetic water. Even got my wife interested in it.

Lew: That is wonderful.

Caller: Yes. I put my feet on that half brick, and the pain goes right away.

Lew: Well, that is wonderful. I'm sure glad to hear that.

Caller: It used to wake me up at night.

Lew: How long did it take before you got the effect?

Caller: Ten – fifteen minutes.

Lew: Is that right? And, you suffered with it for how long?

Caller: About a year.

Lew: Well, I'm glad it's gone. Makes it easier to do your job.

Caller: My wife had pain in her calf, and I said, "Honey, here, put this under your leg."

"Oh, that won't do any good."

"Well, try it any anyway." And she did. The pain in her calf went away.

Lew: Right. I used to have muscle cramps in my legs all the time. It would wake me up. I'd be jumping around trying to get rid of them. Since I've been on a magnetic mattress pad, I haven't had one. Period. Not one night.

Caller: Well, that's probably an excellent investment then.

Lew: All right, sir. Keep up the good work.

Chapter Four

Harmful Force Fields

I was penalized an entire grade in college on a speech I once did. The reason? According to the teacher, I was too lazy to look something up and merely said "statistics show." I would have received an "A" but got a "B" for this reason.

Why was the teacher so strict in this regard? Because this sort of thing is sloppy. It gives the author the opportunity to say anything without anyone being able to check it out. Having said this--I can't quote recent statistics, but I'm sure you will agree that there are many people dying of cancer. The leading cause of cancer is also a matter of opinion. It depends on which article you read or whom you choose to listen to. One of the causes of cancer that hardly anyone is considering is harmful force fields, yet there is a multitude of information that suggest a link to cancer.

Today, society, in general, is extremely prosperous. People living at what is called the poverty level live better than kings did a hundred years ago. We walk into a room and flip the lights on. Lightly touching a button brings us information from the other side of the world or fills the room with symphonic music that a mere hundred years ago was played for royalty only.

Electricity, and the system for delivering electricity, makes all this possible. Electricity has given us great ease of living, great comfort, and great entertainment. It has saved lives and has given us a higher, cleaner standard of living. But, on the other hand, it can be a killer. When we use the term electricity, we are talking about a certain type of force field that can be harnessed to power things. All force fields that lie in this range are called electrical force fields. There is a lot of confusion when it comes to force fields. It seems each body of science has its own definition. On one hand, electrical force fields give us great prosperity, but on the other, they are making us sick and killing us.

That brings up another peculiar phenomenon or irresponsibility and laziness. Just as it is so easy to vaguely talk about some statistic, study, or research without giving proper documentation, we are too lazy to search for answers. Electricity is killing us, and we are too lazy to fix the problem. If you live in a house or work in a place with electricity, you are being bombarded by deadly force fields. Every electrical appliance and every wire with an appliance turned on is emitting a force field. This force field penetrates your body and puts stress on your individual cells and your overall system.

The main reason this force field is dangerous is because it is alternating. When we talk about the alternating characteristic of force fields, we are talking about the direction in which it is spinning. Remember that all force fields travel in circles. When they penetrate your body, they are setting molecules into a spin. They also rearrange molecular structure. An excellent example of a molecule in which the molecular structure is rearranged is the hydrogen molecule. This single molecule is responsible for the acid-alkaline balance in your body.

When this molecule travels through the force field of a properly designed therapeutic magnet, it is rearranged. If it is in such an arrangement to have an acidic pH, its pH will increase. This happens instantly every time. This is demonstrated with a glass of sour grapefruit juice or bitter coffee. Taste the juice or coffee. Then take a properly designed therapeutic magnet and circle it around the outside of the glass or cup about four times. Taste it again. If you can't notice any difference, turn the magnet over and go around in the same direction as before. Now taste it, and it will be wonderfully sweet and flavorful. This is because the pH was instantly elevated. Anyone who has a properly designed therapeutic magnet and a glass of grapefruit juice can do this.

A friendly force field will change the pH in grapefruit juice, coffee, water, or any other liquid, including your blood, almost immediately. This raises another question: If a friendly force field will change liquid for the better, what will an unfriendly force field do?

The answer is that it will cause excessive stress. It will disrupt the distribution system of oxygen and nutrients as well as the elimination system. If the body does not have enough energy at the site where killer force fields are penetrating, the cells will become under nourished, under oxygenated, and over loaded with poisons. The body will do its best to replace cells that need to be replaced, but the new cells will not be healthy. They will be disorganized and sickly. Researchers and other scientific experts call this condition cancer.

Here's what happens: A clockwise spinning force field penetrates your body. Your molecules spin clockwise. A split second later a counter-clockwise force field penetrates your body. Your molecules stop and jerk back to spin the other way. This process is repeated. This process is called alternating. Another term is AC, which stands for alternating current. This jerking and spinning damages the molecules and then the cells. This action is like the agitator in a washing machine. Meanwhile, the body is doing its best to repair the damage. Prolonged exposure to force fields weakens the body. As the body is weakened, it loses its ability to keep up with repairs. The cells become injured and stay that way.

Sometimes the body will build up a shield to protect you. When you notice this shield, it feels like a lump. Most people see a doctor, and the doctor wants to remove it. The body builds up a shield to protect you from killer force fields, and the doctor removes it.

You have the surgery, carry on with your life-style, and go right back to where the killer force fields penetrated your body only to have them penetrate your body again. The body builds its shield back up again. The doctor removes it again. If this has happened to you, or you know of someone it has happened to, study your activities and find the electrical appliance or wire this dangerous force field is coming from.

The doctor may also introduce an extremely dangerous force field called radiation. The concept of radiation is to kill cancerous cells. Unfortunately, many healthy, organized cells are killed too. Before the radiation, that area had at least some good, healthy cells to carry out their function. Now they are gone, and the area screams out for help. This screaming is called pain.

Let's pause a moment and think about the rationale of using radiation. Why do they want to kill the disorganized, sickly cells? They say to keep them from spreading. If the cells are so sick they can't reproduce correctly, how are they going to spread? When the unhealthy cells are killed, it puts enormous stress on the body. This happens because the body now has a huge repair job. The person has reduced energy to function. Those taking radiation treatments sleep a lot and find it very difficult to function. If the body has enough energy to repair the damage, all is well. If it doesn't, the body is further weakened. The real danger starts when the person exposes himself or herself to the same killer force fields that started this process in the first place.

Over time, the body has less and less ability to repair the damage caused by the continued exposure to regular household current. As the situation becomes worse and worse, the screams get louder and louder, which is in the form of pain. What is the answer? When a person is badly laden with disorganized cells, he or she needs extra energy to help the body rebuild them.

Instead of killing cells with radiation, the goal of magnetic therapy is to provide the area with oxygen and nutrients so the cells are replaced with healthy ones. When you place a properly designed therapeutic magnet directly over these cells, the magnet immediately starts to organize them. One by one the molecules become streamlined and healthy and are able to carry out their function. The cell's components become healthy, oxygen and nutrients are delivered and poisons are carried away. As the decayed flesh disappears, pH returns to normal and the body gets better.

One solution to this problem would be to stay out of buildings that are wired for electricity. That is probably not possible, or necessary, if you use properly designed therapeutic magnets.

Here's why. AC current bombards your body all day long. You go to bed with partially stressed, disorganized molecules and cells. When you sleep, your body's main function is to repair and restore the damage caused the day before. If you sleep on a properly designed therapeutic mattress pad, the friendly force fields penetrate your body sending individual molecules into an organizing spin. The pH is set to normal and the body's energy is released to prepare you for an active, productive day. The body has energy to properly nourish your skin so your skin looks healthy and young. The body may have enough energy to heal long-term health problems.

I have deliberately restricted my use of the word "cancer." In fact, I avoid using all of the disease labels. I do not use their names because I don't believe they are correct in their estimation of the symptoms of disease. They search for a cure for diseases but never find one. Yet, if I said that therapeutic magnets would cure their diseases, they would object. With magnetic therapy, we take it one day and one symptom at a time. If one sort of treatment does not seem to be working, we try something else. The great thing is that if we don't get the right treatment the first time, we try not to harm the body further by removing the wrong organ or causing the body needless suffering from side effects.

Allow me to drive this point home. Killer force fields from electrical wires, computer screens, microwaves, and all electrical appliances penetrate the body and disorganize cells, causing the body great stress. Friendly force fields, from properly designed therapeutic magnets, organize them again.

I am questioned frequently about sleeping on a waterbed. In my opinion, it is a death sentence. Why? Since water is an excellent conductor of electricity, it makes alternating force fields more dangerous. I'm sure you have heard the warnings about lightning when it's raining. Go inside. Many golf courses have been closed while they waited for the rain and lightening to quit.

I'm sure you have heard the warnings about using an electrical appliance in the bathtub. If your appliance has any kind of malfunctioning wires and you touch it with wet hands dangerous electrical force fields discharge into you. You probably wouldn't survive if an operating radio or hair dryer fell into the water with you.

The same situation is true with waterbeds. The dangerous force fields come from the waterbed heater. You are sleeping on water and are being penetrated with killer force fields more dangerous than the most powerful high voltage lines. This creates a considerable amount of stress on the body. At night when the body is supposed to repair and rejuvenate itself from the day's activities, all it can do is defend itself from the attack of these force fields.

One way to keep your waterbed and have the best of both worlds is to warm the water before you go to bed; then unplug it. To stay warm have a magnetic mattress pad on it. The magnets act as heat sources to keep you warm. Electric blankets and heating pads are almost as unhealthy as waterbeds. You already know why. You are exposing your body to killer force fields every place it touches. It seems ironic. You have pain, and the painful area responds to warmth. It receives immediate comfort, but long-term damage. We also listed electrical wires as hazardous. The reason we did is because they emit an alternating force field. If you get close enough to "hot" wires, the dangerous force fields will penetrate your body. The closer you are to the source of the force fields and the longer you are exposed, the more harmful it is.

Have you seen products that claim to protect you from these dangerous force fields? Consider this possibility. Recall the force field: It is a spinning spiral. As it leaves the source, it dissipates exponentially if the force field is direct current or unipole. In other words, the spiral is spinning in just one direction.

Alternating force fields do not dissipate that quickly. This is another reason I call them killer force fields. To protect yourself from them, you would have to shield either yourself or each wire and appliance. You would also have to shield the high voltage lines near your house. Wood and rubber act as insulating shields. Most household materials tend to slow the force fields down and insulate to a certain degree.

There is another product that claims to protect people against killer force fields. The strategy is to attract them away from you. This device is a pendant hung from a cord around a person's neck. What kind of a product would be able to accomplish this? Because the north pole is attracted to the south and the south pole is attracted to the north, you would need something with both a north and south pole to attract both poles of the force field. But what about the human body? The human body is a magnet, too, and has a north and a south pole. So, in order for this apparatus to work, its attraction of the north and the south pole must be greater than that of the human body.

To determine if this were effective, you would have to get a meter, stand in front of a microwave, and measure the force field. Then, you would put the pendant on and measure the force field at the pendant and at your body. If it works, any bipolar or alternating magnet would work. Magnetic jewelry would work, too.

Hematite is a natural stone with natural magnetic properties that makes a beautiful black pearl-looking necklace. Companies can magnetize it to the ultimate charge it will accept. If the pendant works to draw force fields away from the body, then so would the hematite necklace.

To summarize: Force fields from household electricity, electrical appliances, and high voltage utility lines travel to penetrate your body. They are alternating, which means they spin one way, then back the other.

This action causes individual molecules to spin one way, jerk to a stop and spin back the other way. They become injured and the body must repair them. When the body runs out of energy, its cells grow disorganized, circulation cannot carry on normally, neighboring cells cannot get oxygen and nutrients, and poisons cannot be hauled away. This is a well-know condition hurting thousands and thousands of people.

Ways to Protect Yourself from Killer Force Fields

- Live and work in a cave with no electricity.
- Insulate all electrical wires and appliances.
- Do research to find ways to effectively shield yourself from these force fields.
- Sleep on a magnetic mattress pad to assist the body in repairing the damage, and wear as many magnetic products as you can to assist the body to repair itself.
- Do not sleep on a waterbed with the heater on.
- Do not use electrical heating pads or blankets.
- Become responsible.

Don't wait for someone to coddle you into taking care of yourself. You don't know all the answers. Search for them.

This is your body. No doctor or anyone else loses more than you if you get sick and even die.

Chapter Five

Germs Are Friends, Not Enemies

We have all heard the saying: "We are digging our own graves with our teeth." But we don't listen to this voice as we enjoy a burger, fries, diet soda, and a piece of pie--popular food in America. Another fact about our situation is, depending on whose statistics you accept, one out of every two people die of heart disease, and one out of every three die of cancer. Many experts say a major reason for this is diet. No. You aren't going to get a lecture on eating right. You already know what food is good for you and what is not. And there are already many good books on nutrition.

The term "couch potato" applies to far too many Americans, mainly because they are watching many hours of television. In fact, Americans often spend as many hours watching television as they do working. Still, we aren't going to waste space in this book telling you to exercise--the media and bookstores are full of information about that.

A leading cause of poor health and disease is a person's *belief* about germs. The following pages will point out why germs are our friends and not our enemies. Disease actually can be a cure, but the popular strategy, at present, for solving the issues of poor health and disease is to kill germs and stop the symptoms of disease. When you have a cold, you sneeze. This is your body's natural way of getting rid of toxin and poison build-up. Yet, you seek medicine that will stop you from sneezing or coughing.

With every natural way of quickly and efficiently ridding the body of poisons, there is a popular strategy to stop it. By stopping the natural out-flowing of bodily fluids loaded with poisons and toxins, you are sabotaging the natural way of getting better.

Everyone agrees that diet and exercise are essential to good health, but a lot of people don't act with what they know. They eat unwholesome food and lie around while the body digests it. As a result, they have no energy for anything else. This contributes to poor health. Most people simply don't realize that germs are their friends and that disease can be a cure.

Recently, there was a garbage strike in New York City. When the workers went on strike, garbage started piling up in the streets, and rats appeared to feed on the rotting garbage. What is the solution to this dilemma? You have two choices--get rid of the rats or eliminate the garbage. If the rats are removed, you still have the garbage. But if we eliminate the garbage, the rats will not have food to eat and will retreat or starve. The same applies to germs. When you feel sick, you have a build-up of garbage in your system, and germs appear to eliminate the garbage.

If you take antibiotics to kill the germs, you still have the garbage and you are still sick. But if you seek to get rid of the garbage, the germs have nothing left to live on and retreat. The real solution to the problem of garbage in the streets was the garbage collectors circulating in their trucks to collect the garbage. The real solution to the problem of poison and toxin build-up in the human body is the lymph system circulating bodily fluids and carrying the garbage away.

Both in the city and in the body, the collection of garbage is an ongoing process. Anywhere trucks can't go, there is a garbage build-up. Similarly, anywhere there is restriction of the lymph system, there is garbage build-up. Germs and rats do their part to carry it away. They only eat garbage. You never find rats in a field or garden eating fresh, clean, good food. They only eat things that are decaying. Likewise, never in the history of medical research has anyone been able to make germ cultures grow in healthy tissue.

In the body, the blood system circulates fuel for metabolism, and the lymph system carries poisons away. Good circulation is a must for both systems. If you eat the right foods and exercise, circulation will improve.

The most underrated strategy for improving circulation is Magnetic Therapy. You place a properly designed therapeutic magnet on your body, and the force fields penetrate your flesh. All force fields travel in spiraling circles. These circles cause molecules in your body to spin, and when cells spin, they become streamlined. Streamlined components circulate better than jagged, odd-shaped components, and better circulation allows the body to better eliminate poisons and toxins.

Good health begins with individual cells. Each cell is a manufacturing plant that carries out a specific function as well as making adenosine triphosphate (ATP), which fuels the body. A retail store is a great example of different teams working together. Stores grouped together are called a market. The market place functions just like the body, with some participants manufacturing things, others distributing things, others cleaning, and still others doing many additional things. Cells in your body also work together. They all have their specific duties as an individual, yet they are all members of a special team that works together. As the distribution system is vital for a marketplace to function, circulation is vital for cells to work together and function. Oxygen is one of the things that must circulate freely in order for cells to do their work. When the delivery of oxygen is stopped, or even restricted, the cell suffers and sometimes dies. Cells cannot live without oxygen, so if the oxygen they need is not delivered, they cannot do their best work.

Magnetic force fields penetrating any area help improve circulation so cells receive the oxygen they need, and as these cells use oxygen to convert into ATP, waste products are eliminated. Proper circulation to eliminate these waste products is very important. The very second that circulation is slowed, waste products begin to build up, smothering the cell in its own waste. Unless these poisons are carried away, the cell will poison itself and die. When the cell dies, the circulatory system now has an entire cell to carry away, and if the circulation system is restricted, the dead cell cannot be moved and begins to decay. This puts an even greater burden on the circulatory system.

When the garbage isn't carried away through normal channels and begins to decay and build up, other mechanisms step in to assist. These mechanisms are called symptoms of disease: sneezing, coughing, indigestion, sweating, pain and shortness of breath, just to name a few. They could manifest themselves as a fever, for when things get warm, they move faster. Fever warms the body and the fluids flow more freely. This is one reason why it is important to do as your Aunt Mary used to say: "Eat your hot chicken soup, and let the fever run its course."

Germs may appear as the rats did in New York City. As soon

as they consume the garbage, circulation is restored. Without them, the garbage stays right where it is to drown the cells in their own waste and restrict circulation. This garbage may begin to ooze through the pores in the skin. The pores grow bigger, so more garbage can be eliminated, and redness may develop as if the skin were being stretched. The skin may itch or blisters may form. Unpleasant as it may sound, this is a natural process to eliminate poisons. Placing a therapeutic magnet directly over this eruption assists the body in restoring circulation, so garbage can be whisked away through the regular elimination system. So avoid treating the skin with astringents, which restricts the pores, making it more difficult for poisons to get through.

The Germ Theory

Someone has a cold and sneezes on you--and now you have a cold. Why? According to the usual theory, germs from the sneeze enter your body, attack it, reproduce and continue to hurt you. But this scenario makes sense only when you ignore the scientific facts.

Germs, whether you call them bacteria, virus, molds, or yeast, do not attack healthy tissue! It has NEVER been demonstrated in a laboratory. This belief that germs are the cause of disease has created an entire body of medicine which is in search of this cause. It has created an entire industry to track down germs and eliminate them. Doctors marvel when new, more resilient strains come into existence, and researchers struggle to develop new antibiotics to kill them. An entire body of medicine searches for the cure for germ-causing diseases.

Scientifically there are two theories. One says that germs are friends, and the other, more popular theory, says germs are enemies. Both theories can't be right. The germ theory is questioned by some of experts. Stanley L. Robbins, M.D., a professor of pathology at the Harvard Medical School, in his

Robbins Pathologic Basis of Disease, asked the question: "Is a 'single cause' of a disease an accurate evaluation in light of today's understandings?" This expert doesn't think so. Why? Because in some studies, people and animals were deliberately infected with the same germs, yet they all didn't develop the same disease. Nor did the ones who did develop it do so at the same rate or with the same degree of severity. Researchers have repeated experiments like this in laboratories over and over again, only to get the same results. The simple fact that certain germs or viruses are present does not mean a person has a certain disease. The level of toxicity in the body and the symptoms it manifests will determine the disease and its severity—not the germs and virus trying to decontaminate it.

Koch's Postulates

Nobel Prize winner Robert Koch lists four criteria to determine whether a disease is contagious and caused by a particular germ or virus (microbe). These are called Koch's Postulates:

> *1) If germs cause disease, they must be found in every single case in which a certain set of symptoms is called a certain disease.*

They are not. It is a well-known fact that a disease may arise in the absence of the germ that is supposed to cause it. If the rats caused the garbage strike, why weren't there tons of rats on the street before the garbage strike. If germs caused the disease, why weren't they present at the start of the disease?

> *2) If germs cause disease, they must never be found apart from the disease.*

If rats caused the garbage strike, then every place there are rats, there must be a garbage strike. Germs of pneumonia, tuberculosis, and diphtheria are often found in perfectly healthy people who do not have these diseases. The germs cannot be the cause unless every single time they are present, the disease which they are supposed to cause must be present. Just as rats are often found where there is no garbage strike, germs are found where there is no disease.

3) If germs cause disease, they will attack healthy tissue.

In order for germs to live and reproduce, they must have unhealthy, decaying tissue. This has been demonstrated over and over again in laboratories. Scientists cannot grow a culture of germs unless they have decaying tissue because germs simply will not grow in healthy tissue.

4) If germs cause disease, it must be possible to take certain germs causing a certain disease and inject them into another person, causing that person to have that same disease.

In 1921, scientists conducted experiments with 62 volunteers. The objective of this experiment was to cause a certain disease with the germ that was supposed to cause it. They injected the germs into the volunteers, sprayed them on their food and directly through their open mouths into their throats--some got the disease--some did not. The result of the experiment was that there was no discernible reaction. The researchers concluded that if certain germs cause certain diseases, then they should cause those diseases, and only those diseases, every single time. A cause must be constant and specific in its influence or it is not a cause. To this, I would like to add two Lyon Postulates. In making the comparison with such a great scientist and researcher as Dr. Koch, I am in no way putting myself on his level. I have tremendous respect for a person who would "break ranks" with political pressure to fall in line. I also admire the Nobel Prize process for these same reasons.

Lyon's Postulates

1) Using weapons to kill the scavengers is not effective because the scavengers are not the problem.

There are weapons that kill rats--rat poison, traps, bullets. If these weapons work, and they do, all you have to do is use these weapons to get rid of the rats. In the garbage strike, these weapons were used, but unfortunately, they were used on things that they weren't intended for. Children got into the rat poison, bullets missed and hit something else, and traps caught house-hold pets. But these are just side effects. To the extent the weapons were used, the rats died. But the garbage remained. But let's say they were successful and killed all the rats. Then other scavengers stepped up to carry the garbage away. Anyway, the rats got stronger and became resistant to the poisons.

Researchers created improved poisons, better bullets and traps, and the rats became stronger and outsmarted their enemies again. A vicious cycle begins, and the end result is: You can't kill all of the rats all of the time. Poison may kill rats in the laboratory, traps may work some of the time, and bullets may work some of the time. But there is no weapon that will kill all the scavengers all of the time. But what is our goal here? *To eliminate the waste.*

There is a weapon that kills germs--antibiotics. If this weapon works, all we have to do is use it to eliminate germs. In the case of a cold, these weapons are used and will continue to be used because they work.

Unfortunately, these weapons are used on things that they were not intended for. Friendly germs and other microbes are killed also. This overloads the lymph system with additional waste to carry away and slows its circulation even more. Other mechanisms of the body step in to try to assist, perhaps with a fever, and more medicine is used to fight the fever. Again, good germs die along with the so-called bad ones, and the effectiveness of the lymph system is even more obstructed. But these are just side effects. To the extent the weapons were used, the poisons died. But the garbage remained. Again, let's say they were successful and killed all the germs. Other scavengers stepped in to carry the garbage away. The germs got stronger and became resistant to the antibiotics, and researchers created improved antibiotics. The germs became stronger and outsmarted them again. The vicious cycle begins, and the end result is: You can't kill all of the germs all of the time. There is no weapon that will kill all scavengers all the time.

2) If germs cause disease and antibiotics kill germs, then properly employing the right weapon would kill the germs, thus eliminating the disease.

But this doesn't happen. Frequently, doctors will prescribe an antibiotic that kills germs, but the disease remains. In a reexamination of the culture, the doctors find that the germs are still alive and well. So, to remedy the situation, the doctors will prescribe a larger dose to be taken more frequently, and the reexamination of the culture shows that the germs the antibiotic was trying to kill are gone. Yet, the patients still have the disease, or they are better. If germs were the cause, and the antibiotic successfully killed the germs, then the patients would get better every single time.

In order for this process to be truly scientific, the results must be reproducible in every single case. If it fails just one time, it is no longer scientific but is a matter of hit or miss.

Medical experts say there is a huge variety of germs in everyone's system, yet we obviously don't have all the diseases they say these germs cause.

Germs do not attack healthy tissue or cause disease any more than rats cause a garbage build-up.

Then *why* do we get sick? What is the cause of disease? It is my position that sickness and disease have one and only cause: poor circulation.

Poor Circulation Can Be Brought On By Stress

When people get upset, they become tense. Right before your eyes, the muscles tighten, making it more difficult for blood to travel through. It also makes it harder for the lymph system to carry poison away. To the exact degree of your stress, circulation is restricted, and to the exact degree of restriction, poisons build up. To the exact degree of build-up, these poisons look for alternative methods to get out, and these methods are called symptoms of disease, which can be one or many.

Established medicine labels this collection of symptoms a certain disease.

What are these symptoms? There are only a few. A certain symptom can be found in different places with different severity but still remains the same symptom.

Symptoms Of Disease And Poisoning

Fever	Chills	Sweating
Fatigue	Malaise	Skin Irritation
Anorexia	Throat Irritation	Headache
Weakness	Cough	Nasal Discharge
Impaired Breathing	Diarrhea	Constipation
Nausea	Vomiting	Muscle Pain
Urinary Difficulties	Eye Irritations	Photophobia
Paresis	Paralysis	Weight Loss
Inflamed Lymph Nodes	Weight Gain	Joint Pain
Lesions	Infection	Irritability
Delirium	Chemical Imbalance	Shaking

The symptoms of disease and poisoning are the same, and every one of these symptoms is caused by poor circulation. If you place a properly designed therapeutic magnet directly over the area where there is a symptom, circulation can be restored and the symptom can depart. As a result, cells get the necessary nutrients to carry out their functions.

Then the whole body functions normally. Poor circulation can be caused by stress, from changes in the weather, or by a change in the seasons because your body is striving to keep you warm and does not have enough energy to properly maintain itself. Before I learned about therapeutic magnets, I endured a cold every fall season.

If you take a moment, you will notice most people that live in areas where there are seasons also develop colds and flu. Why? Getting cold could be one reason. When the body is cold, it strives to get warm to maintain its standard 98.6 body temperature.

The brain, working together with the body, does its part in creating desires to eat warm food, such as hot chocolate, chili, or soup. These foods help the body stay warm temporarily. But, in the long term, these foods congest the system, reducing circulation, and, therefore, putting even more stress on an already stressed body.

As the debris in the system builds up, pressure is created, and the poisons expel themselves any way they can, such as sneezing, coughing or vomiting.

Poor Circulation Can Be Caused By the Expectation of Sickness

For example, we are conditioned to expect sickness by the news media and our new seasons——Flu and Cold. Many people expect to get sick, and sure enough, they do.

The mind systematically shuts down circulation, and the person becomes genuinely sick. However, some people or doctors have found a strategy to get the mind to heal itself.

Poor Circulation Can Be Caused By the Same Vaccine Used to Prevent the Illness

In his book entitled *Emerging Viruses, AIDS and Ebola,* Dr. Len Horowitz demonstrates to the logical, non-political mind that vaccines do not prevent disease, never have, and never will. Where do vaccines come from?

The manufacturing of vaccines is one of the most disgusting processes you can imagine. For one vaccine, scientists shave a calf's stomach and cut into its skin with razors. Without bandages or any effort to heal the calf, it is left for approximately three days.

By this time the cuts are oozing pus, feverish, swollen and very sore. The calf is then strapped to a table and the pus, scabs and other substances are scraped from the sores.

These substances are then strained, stirred and further processed, and this putrefying, disgusting, filthy stuff is injected into the blood stream of healthy human babies, children, and adults. This vaccine clogs the circulation process, and if the body already has a circulation problem, disease may result.

Poor Circulation Can Be Caused By Diet

Rich, fatty, dense foods make the body work harder to break them down for use. Remember the body does not have unlimited energy, and if the body does not have the energy to properly digest and change the food into energy, then it becomes a burden to the system.

If the body does not have the ability to flush this newly created poison out through the lymph system, it rots and decays right where it is. The cells that were counting on this new delivery for materials to carry out their jobs must compensate and make do with what they have. The glow of health fades.

Poor Circulation Can Be Caused By Reduced Activity

Computer operators and programmers work harder with their minds than almost anyone. They can move mountains with a single keystroke, and they must accomplish more than some other occupations. But because their work does not require them to be on their feet and move around, the muscles are not much used. Because these muscles are not used, they start to decline and shrink. There is a saying: "If you don't use it, you lose it." Muscles are huge consumers of energy, burning a considerable amount of fat, even while you sleep. If a person eats the same amount and type of food, while at the same time reducing activity, thus not using muscles, it puts additional stress on the system. Because the system is stressed and cannot transform all the unnecessary food into energy, the so-called half-used food is converted to fat.

Excessive fat blocks the natural paths of circulation, and the cells in that area become oxygen starved. The pH decreases, and a person's energy level deteriorates. Without proper amounts of oxygen, cells cannot reproduce properly and become disorganized. Any area of physical weakness is weakened even more, and the body's level of health decreases. Exercise is the fastest way to rinse out the system. Just as our bodies need to sweat to function properly, plain, clear water is the best way to clean anything.

However, I know of several examples of elderly people who sleep on magnetic mattress pads, sit on magnetic cushions all day, wear magnetic insoles in their shoes and they are just as healthy as if they were exercising and sweating.

As much as I am a proponent for therapeutic magnets, I am a bigger proponent for doing things the way God intended. I would never suggest that magnets will replace a natural function like exercise.

Poor Circulation Can Be Caused By Chemical Imbalance

This could be anything from excess chemicals in your drinking water to an ingredient in your shampoo. Anytime the body has to divert energy away from normal functions, the circumstance is created for poison build up, and, therefore, disease.

In alternative medicine circles, saying the word "cure" is lethal. To put it in simple, direct terms, the use of that word is completely unnecessary. Using the word "cure" is not only unnecessary but also irrelevant. So, we who use magnetic therapy, step up and out of the dead-end streets. We follow the rules that have been in place for hundreds and thousands of years. The practice of exploring dead-end streets looking for germs to kill has failed. We set a new standard, the standard God intended–perfect health.

Yeast and Fungus

Other microscopic organisms, yeast, molds, and fungi assist the decaying process. According to most doctors, the majority of diseases are caused by bacteria, viruses, and other germs in the same category. No one has been considering yeast, molds, and fungi, except Dr. Robert O. Young.

I met Mr. Young in Kona, Hawaii, last year. The Youngs and their team had designed a system to analyze an individual's blood right before one's eyes. The lab technician pricked my finger ever so slightly to get a tiny spot of blood; then he placed it on a slide and put it under a microscope.

Together we examined it and looked at a number of things to determine what areas should be focused on. We looked at the space between the blood cells, for if there is enough space, the cells can properly circulate. If they are clustered, they can still circulate, but not as well as they could, and as a result, will not deliver oxygen and other nutrients to the cells efficiently. We looked at the shape of the cell, which should be round. If they are jagged, oval, or any other shape, circulation cannot be completely efficient. Then we looked at parasites in the blood. The main parasites we were looking for were yeast and molds. This is where I depart from Dr. Young in regard to his medical strategy, which is exactly the same as the rest of the doctors looking for scavengers. If there is yeast in the blood, then it has a purpose, just like germs. The real problem is the waste build up that is obstructing proper circulation. If you kill the yeast, you still have the garbage. The focus should be on improving circulation. When the garbage is dealt with by the body, the scavengers do not have enough food and disappear.

In case you are interested, my blood was in great shape. I have been sleeping on a magnetic mattress pad for a number of years, sit on a magnetic cushion on my office chair and in the car, and I have magnetic insoles in every pair of shoes I wear. My blood is continuously in a properly designed magnetic force field and, as a result, is in excellent condition.

Mr. Young states in his company's pamphlet *Innerlight, The Bodycology System and Diet*: "The road toward understanding the process of restoring health has been a long one. Many enemies have been identified: germs, viruses, bacteria, and even yeast. Entire schools of science have been established upon each of these. But these are just pieces of a larger puzzle. In the early seventies, scientists began recognizing the role yeast, such as Candida Albicans, play[s] in illness. Best-selling books (most notably, William Crook's *The Yeast Connection*) touted anti-yeast diets and medications to control the Candida yeast.

Dr. Orian Truss published a book called *The Missing Diagnosis* in which he stated his conclusion that yeast is implicated in a wide variety of conditions, from depression to allergies. More pieces of the puzzle were revealed in the late eighties. Distinguished research scientist Mr. Robert O. Young, Ph.D.,

D.Sc., is recognized throughout the world as the man who has described a new paradigm of human disease. Understanding the role yeast and fungus play in illness, Dr. Young blended his years of exhaustive research with decades of published research and clinical studies to finally piece together the pathways to both illness and wellness, outlined in Innerlight's "The Cycle of Imbalance," and "The Cycle Of Balance" chart. There is only one disease—the constant over[-] acidification of the blood and tissues. This disturbs the central regulation of the human body, unbalancing it."

I tend almost to agree with this last statement. The reason I believe it is when the blood, or any other circulating bodily fluid, does not circulate freely, there is a build-up of poisons. The natural pH of poison is low, or acidic. If the blood and tissues are acidic, then there is poor circulation, which is indicated by low pH.

In Conclusion

Researchers and scientists have been searching for a cure for diseases by searching for the enemy and killing it. This research has been going on for decades and has cost hundreds of millions of dollars. It has become an endless loop. The moment they think they have discovered a cure, some outside influence they didn't consider enters the scene. However, magnetic therapy demonstrates incredible success. The ways to use magnets seem almost endless. Because it is so safe, everyone can be a researcher discovering breakthrough scientific information that will help people today and for generations to come. When you step back and see all the technologies working together, you see huge potential. Properly designed therapeutic magnets increase the effectiveness of every therapy, and the levels of health we can achieve are UNLIMITED!

Chapter Six

Is It Really All in Your Mind?

It's true, you know. You are sick because you have made yourself sick in your mind. You are healthy because you have made yourself healthy in your mind. We really can, and do, live a life of Heaven or Hell in our minds. The working of the mind influences the effectiveness of magnetic therapy. A good, solid belief in magnetic therapy makes it work better. On the other hand, a skeptical, fearful, negative belief does not keep it from working—but it does keep the user from realizing that it worked. The person gets better but gives the credit to something else and then quits using the magnets and grows worse. Clearly, magnetic therapy is no exception to the old saying: "It's all in your mind." In other words, if you believe in magnetic therapy, it helps. But even if you don't, it still works. However, if you are against it and don't believe in magnetic therapy, you are slowing the healing process.

I know of case after case where people were being helped and just simply would not believe it. They experienced themselves getting better; they saw the results with their own eyes, yet they gave the credit to other things. These "things" had failed them time and time again, but instead of giving the magnets credit, they gave credit to these past failures. They quit using the magnets because it is inconvenient to strap a magnet to your body. Naturally, their original symptoms returned; they suffered, and some even died--all because they would not believe in magnetic therapy, even though they saw it working with their own eyes.

There are hundreds of articles and books discussing and explaining this phenomena; however, hardly anyone is talking about magnetic therapy. Because the mind is vital to good health, I want to give some examples: I've heard of the mind dissolving tumors, that the mind is more powerful than the influence of drugs, and that the mind causes a person to be fat or thin.

Many people are striving for wealth and prosperity in the wrong places, while the real answers lie in the recesses of their minds, commonly referred to as our beliefs.

Our beliefs cause us to live a joyous, fulfilled life as if we are in Heaven, but they also create a dim, desperate life as if we are in Hell. Unfortunately, this statement "It's all in your mind" is becoming a "cop-out," and is spoken more and more by doctors when they cannot find a reason for a patient's disease and pain.

The biggest travesty is a doctor telling a person it is all in his or her mind, and then walking out, never to schedule another appointment with the patient. If the doctor is right and it is all in the patients' minds, then why didn't the doctor help them heal those minds to make them better?

In my business, I hear people complaining about doctors constantly. They complain that they cut out the wrong kidney, prescribed the wrong drug or combination of drugs, or talked them into having surgery. They complain about and blame doctors mercilessly. But these people are not prisoners who are forced to do anything. Before every surgery, the person signs his or her name consenting to it. With every prescription, the person must travel to the drug store, ask for it, and pay for it— none of these steps are forced upon that person.

They know up front that doctors are people and that people make mistakes. If they cut out the wrong kidney, it is terrible, but the person knew his or her fate was in hands of someone else. People ignore the fact that it is their body, and they are the ones who gain--and the ones who suffer. Each of us is responsible. Each person must become his or her own doctor.

Consider it. Who knows exactly how you feel? You do. Who knows, without looking anything up, what medicine you are taking to avoid drugs reacting adversely with each other? You do.

Who knows your body's exact response to different foods or drugs? You do. Because you are the best person to make the diagnosis, you are the best person to prescribe the treatment. You are intelligent. If anyone can learn it, you can; and you can find the time. It takes more time to keep a doctor's appointment and wait than it probably would to get on the Internet and search out the facts needed to make your decision on how to treat yourself.

I recently went to a structural therapist, and his secretary had me complete a medical history form. All these forms are basically alike. They ask who my doctor is, and I answered "Self." I listen to what these doctors and therapists have to say; and if it doesn't make sense, then I get all the facts, investigate further, and decide for myself what to do regarding my health. If I make a mistake, I don't blame anyone. I have respect for doctors and other experts in the healthcare field, and I admire them for their great accomplishments in getting a college degree. But my respect is not blind, nor does it elevate to the level of worship.

Let's Hear It from the Animals

I had a wonderful friend—a German Shepherd named Dillinger. He was born in the summer, but on Thanksgiving of that same year, there was a knock on our door, early in the morning while it was still dark. My son Jack went to answer the door, and standing there was a hunter, and the hunter informed Jack that he had shot one of our dogs. We scrambled into our clothes to go outside and find out which dog was shot, physically locate the wounded animal, and help him. Jack discovered that Dillinger was missing, and we were even more determined to find him. As we searched, shots were fired over our heads. When it started to snow, and all tracks and signs of blood were covered, we decided it was hopeless and gave up.

Bitter cold set in over the next few days, and a week came and went. We had given up all hope that Dillinger had survived. Then, on the following Monday morning, Jack went out to take care of the dogs and horses. It was dark, and I was preparing breakfast in the kitchen. "Mom! You'd better come out here." The expression in his voice caused me to drop what I was doing to go and see what he was talking about. Reduced to little more than skin and bones and dragging one of his back legs, there was Dillinger! I greeted him as a long-lost friend. I thought quickly, "This dog has been without food and water for about ten days, and he is going to endure more trauma in surgery. We are going to take him to the vet to do everything we can to save his life. I really love this dog."

I can remember my inner dialog as if it were yesterday. "He is going to be operated on in about two hours; he is going to need everything possible to get him through. He is in bad shape, and he needs strength. Therefore, he needs to eat now. In about two hours, this food will be supplying his body with the energy he needs to pull through." I opened the refrigerator and got out everything I thought he would eat and gobble up quickly. I knew he wouldn't eat his dog food, so I gave him a big bowl of raw eggs and leftover goulash. It worked. He devoured it.

We scrambled to get ready and loaded Dilly into the back seat of our car. It was still dark when we got to the vet. We carried the dog in and put him on the stainless steel examination table where he lay seemingly lifeless. "This dog is pretty far gone. I don't think he can withstand surgery," said Dr. Madison. I responded, "Do what you can. I really like this dog." Dillinger was nearing total unconsciousness.

There was nothing more for us to do, so we left. I was a student at the local technical school then, so I went to school and forced myself to keep my mind on my studies. Noon came and I finally had a break to call the veterinary clinic. "Is Dillinger still breathing?" I asked. "Yes," answered the receptionist. I made arrangements to stop and see him on my way home. A confident, grateful feeling came over me.

Around five o'clock, I entered the clinic and was escorted to the cages where they kept animals recovering from one procedure or another. The attendant told me that Dilly was still unconscious from the surgery removing his leg. They really didn't expect him to make it, but he was still breathing. I went back again expecting the worst, and there he was lying apparently lifeless in a cage. Then I spoke his name, and he got up! No one could believe it. Then he drank some water. He was going to make it! I sat with him for a few minutes. Finally I told him to go back to sleep and that I would see him in the morning.

From that point on, he was allowed to come in the house. From time to time we would let other pets come in, but Dillinger was the one in charge. He assigned himself the position of caretaker and guard. He took his position very seriously and never played. Months passed. Winter came and went, and still another winter came. The family was doing their usual routine. My mother had come to visit. Our children had become responsible adults, making their own living.

On one particular day we noticed an unusual smell in our house. I thought it peculiar, but as always, I was in a hurry and ignored it. A couple of hours later, we noticed smoke in the hall. Fire had started in the hot water heater, and by the time we found it, the wall and ceiling insulation were in flames. We called the fire department, and they were there in minutes, but the house went fast.

As a result, we moved closer to town with Dilly. A couple of years went by. We had been in the industrial magnet business but now turned our focus to manufacturing therapeutic magnetic products. Nothing happens until something is sold, and to sell products, you must go where the people are. So we decided to take a trip of the southern United States where many people had gone to live in the warmer weather for the winter. We bought a 29-foot trailer to live in, outfitted our car to pull it, loaded up Dilly in the back seat, and took off for Florida. It was a successful selling trip, and we repeated it the next year.

Dilly was eight the first year we toured the South and was getting up in years--approaching the upper life span for German Shepherds. The missing leg was one of the back ones. Big dogs, and especially German Shepherds, have a tendency to have hip problems, and poor Dilly only had one hip to carry the full weight of his near-100-pound body. He seemed to get along fine but was slowing down. The next year we were invited to the home of Pam and Jed. Pam loved Dilly, and he loved her. She invited him into her house, almost as an honored guest, and we stayed about a week, visiting during the days.

During that visit, Pam shamed me with her observation that Dilly needed pain relief and extra help more than anyone else in our family and that he was the only one of us who did not use the therapeutic magnets. I vainly explained that there was such a demand for my time and our products, that every time I started to make him a magnetic pad, we would get an order for one, and it would have to be shipped. The demand on my time was such that I was working twelve hours a day in the business, doing the normal meal preparation and house maintenance, doing the laundry, and excuses, excuses, and more excuses. After all, I was on the road. I couldn't do anything about it now.

When I walked Dilly, we would go about half a block, and he would have to sit down and rest. He was in pain, and I was ignoring it. After a couple of weeks, we settled down for the month of December in Spring Hill, Florida. The second day I was there, I gathered materials and made Dilly a magnetic pet pad. After the very first night he slept on it, I noticed the difference in his body strength. We went for a walk the next morning, and he didn't have to stop to rest!

Dilly's magnetic pet pad turned back the clock. He became a young vibrant dog again and chased rabbits every chance he got. He wanted to go for twice as many walks. It was incredible seeing such a burst of energy when he seemed so elderly just a few weeks earlier.

One night he was asleep in the hallway, and unfortunately, in the middle of the night Lew tripped and stepped on his one back leg. The next morning Little Dilly couldn't walk. I had to carry him outside that morning, and I put him on his magnetic pet pad positioning the injury on the magnets.

We expected he would be in the same condition for several days, but when Lew came home that night, Dilly met him at the door! That night he walked on his own when we went for a walk! When you see miracles like this, a part of you really doesn't believe, so the thought crossed my mind that Dilly was really not that bad in the first place. Then I considered—how many animals do you know that would let someone struggle carrying them everywhere when they are consumed with the desire to get out and run around? None. Animals may decide they like the attention, but the minute they get outside, they lose their focus. They see the grass, smell the scents, hear the sounds, and want to go investigate the smells around the bushes and trees. Dilly was really hurt. Without the magnets, he would have been laid up for at least a week. It was a miracle, but miracles were happening all the time.

The faster you expose an injury to healing force fields, the faster the injury will heal and the faster the pain will go away. Maybe it's all in your head. But then again, maybe it's not. If you think the healing action is all in a person's head, then what about Little Dilly? Did he know anything about magnets when he was placed on a different pad? Did he expect to get almost instant relief? No. Animals accept whatever they get, and they live without questions and complaint. They are never surprised because they don't contemplate what to expect. They are perfect specimens to determine whether or not magnets relieve pain because they are so truthful.

One evening I noticed a tense expression on Little Dilly's face, so I felt his head and it was feverish. I keep a First Aid magnet handy at all times and placed it right between his eyes and kept it there for about 60 seconds. About an hour later, I noticed his tense, painful expression was gone. I felt his head, and it was normal.

The second year we went south, we had a show in St. Paul, Minnesota. The weekend before we were scheduled to leave, Little Dilly had a bad infestation of fleas. We took him to the kennel where he would be staying for a flea bath. This was on Friday afternoon, and we were scheduled to pick him up after five on Sunday. We waited until five and went after him. Lew could not believe the dog he picked up. Little Dilly was dying:

His breath was getting shallow, his body temperature was cooling, and he was getting stiff. The first thing I did when I saw the kind of condition he was in was to hug him and love him. Then I got his magnetic pet pad and slid him on it, and to everyone's amazement, he was warm in twenty minutes! In another twenty minutes, he was drinking water. He was going to make it! It took about six months for a full recovery but a full recovery it was! What had happened? We could only surmise. Maybe it was the poison in the flea dip. Maybe he was miserable about being left in an unfamiliar house and lost hope that he would ever see me again. Perhaps both.

By this time Dilly was over eleven years old, but acted like a puppy at times. He was extremely happy and never irritable. We always knew when he slept on his magnetic pet pad and when he didn't. His energy level was the proof. There were times when he would hurt one of his legs, and it would swell. I would put a magnetic ankle or magnetic wrist wrap directly over the swelling, and to my great surprise, he would actually leave it there.

If I would bandage an open wound, he would promptly chew on the bandage until it came off, but the therapeutic magnets, he left in place. Within a couple of hours, the swelling would usually be gone, but sometimes there were injuries that I didn't notice right away. Those took longer to heal, but every single time, they healed faster than I expected.

Animals have keen instincts. When they are sick, they will find a cool, dark place to lie. They will dig down deeper into the earth. Why? To get out of the sun because the sun's energy is not healing energy. Digging places them in a more intense force field from the earth. There are two scientific concepts that animals understand. The first is that force fields travel more efficiently through solids. The second is the more intense the force field, the faster the healing.

Let me explain the first: Force fields travel more efficiently through solids. Have you ever tried to hear a conversation in a room with the door closed? You placed your ear right up against the door, and what happened? You could hear better. Sound waves and force fields are the same in this regard. The closer you get to the magnet, the stronger the circuit formed for the energies to travel, and you get a more intense force field.

By the way, for this very reason, it is dangerous to sleep on a waterbed with an electric heater, because the water puts you in a more intense force field. The same goes for an electric heating pad or an electric blanket. These electric items, together with their design, expose the body to an intense force field of dangerous, destructive, cancer-causing energy.

Allow me to explain number two: The more intense the force field, the faster the healing. As the force field leaves the power source, the energies disintegrate exponentially. This is simple: The closer you are to the magnet, the more intense the force fields are. The earth is a big magnet, and that's why animals dig to get closer to the source of this healing energy. For those of you who own dogs or cats that you absolutely adore, while it is not easy, if you want the best for your pets, you will allow them to have a dark place on the ground where they can dig. The earth's healing energy helps circulation, and increased circulation gives better health. It provides more energy, a beautiful coat, a happy spirit, and stronger bones, to name a few benefits. But if you can't provide such a place, the next best thing is to provide your pet with a properly designed magnetic pet pad. At thirteen, Little Dilly had a beautiful coat, very little gray on his muzzle, strong white teeth, and eyes which were sparkling and clear. Even though he had only one hip, there was no sign of hip problems, and his hearing had not diminished.

At thirteen, he had the body of a three-year-old. This testimony of health was completely the result of therapeutic magnets. He did not make regular trips to a vet, and he did not have a special diet. Nor did he take vitamins. In fact, we gave him snacks from everything we ate.

When my friend Pam shamed me into putting Little Dilly on a pet pad, his health was probably starting to deteriorate. Thanks to Pam, the magnets gave us about five extra years of love, joy, and happiness with Dilly. Yes, happiness. Little Dilly made us happy. When Lew and I would be having a conversation, and our emotion caused us to raise our voices, Little Dilly would start to get scared, thinking we were going to get mad and argue. He would sidle up to the one who was the most passionate and smile. Lew or I would forget our outburst and smile and pet him. The momentum toward a fight was interrupted, and we were redirected to happiness and love.

On December 3, 1998, Dillinger quit breathing. His system had been shutting down for about a month. It had became harder and harder for him to go for a walk, but he steeled himself with every amount of strength he had and did it. One day, after the morning walk, he could hardly move, and we knew the end was near.

We did not take him to a vet. We decided to love him and keep him comfortable. I made sure he had the most powerful pet pad available at all times. It gave him comfort, and probably a little more time. On December 1, we arrived in Sedona, Arizona. We had a company convention planned.

We had planned to stay the whole month of December and enjoy the more powerful force fields there. Little Dilly was getting weaker and weaker. The next day he jerked himself up and went for a walk almost like normal, but he didn't get far. His strength gave out, and I had to carry him back. I laid him outside where I thought he would be comfortable. He was getting so weak that I said goodbye to him. The sun went down, and he was still alive.

It was not easy, but I carried him inside. He was alive, but getting cold. He was so heavy I barely got up the steps. He lay on the floor between the driver and passenger seats of our new coach, and he didn't want to leave. Lying down beside him, I told him he was a good boy—and that it was OK to die. Then I petted him and hugged him for the last time. But life goes on, and dinner had to be made. Dilly struggled once in a while and tried to get up. Finally a couple of hours later, Lew noticed that Dilly had quit breathing. It is hard to lose your best friend.

I thought back over his life and recalled that his body language was exactly the same four years ago when Pam shamed me into providing a magnetic pet pad for him. Pam sensed and told me that he was not well. His system was shutting down back then. Pam saw it and was courageous enough to say so. That pet pad turned his life around, and except for the last month, he enjoyed those extra years in great happiness. I took him with me everywhere. Where the car went, he went.

Therapeutic magnets made his life comfortable—this German Shepherd had no hip problems, even though his entire body weight had to be carried on one hip. He had all his teeth. His dedication and friendship for me was legendary. Someone said, "It is better to have loved and lost than never to have loved at all." When someone loses a loved one (even an animal) or fails in business or marriage, she or he usually resolves never to try again. Not me. Life is about living and dying. In fact, that is a law of nature. The second we are born, we begin to die. Millions of cells in our bodies die every day. Friends die, but our loving memory of them lives on. We live on.

We heard another pet story from a woman who told us about her dog and cat. These two so-called enemies got along well and had a mutual respect for each other. Each one had its own territory, and the other would not try to invade it. When the lady's cat started limping with joint pain, she bought the cat a magnetic mattress; the magnetic mattress pad relieved the cat's pain, and she quit limping the very first day of owning it.

It is hard to imagine what goes on the minds of animals, but the dog then started invading the cat's territory by trying to get on the pet pad. The next thing she knew, they were fighting over it! So the lady got another pet pad for the dog, and now they are back to respecting each other's territory, each sleeping on its own magnetic pet pad. You have to wonder how the animals knew. How did the dog know about the healing, strengthening energies coming from the mattress pad? How did he know it was beneficial? Because animals use their instincts more than people.

Large dogs like Dillinger, who have hip weaknesses, respond well to magnets. In fact, I have never seen it fail. Within a few hours, a dog that barely walks is noticeably better. For example, one dog we knew had cataracts. The owners placed a large therapeutic magnet in her bed, and they made sure that every time she was in her bed, she had her head positioned on the magnet with her eyes as close as possible to the magnet's north pole. In about six weeks, she had no symptoms of vision loss.

No chapter about animals being helped through magnetic therapy would be complete without telling about Lucky Wedgeworth of Spring Hill, Florida. The following is an excerpt taken from a newsletter entitled the *Lyon Letter # 7.*

DQ?

On our 1996 marketing tour, we were not only doing shows but were also working with team members. Christmas found us in Spring Hill, Florida. Chuck and Dolores Wedgeworth invited us to their home for Christmas dinner, and we met Lucky. Chuck is a good friend of the Stones, who are members of our marketing team. When Bob Stone first told Chuck about medical magnets, he thought it was preposterous that a magnet could do everything Bob said it would. Bob explained that these magnets from Lyons are not just ordinary magnets. Medical magnets are different from ordinary magnets in a number of ways. We have learned how to focus magnetic energy. Medical magnets have the right focus for the area on the body they are trying to affect. Medical magnets are the right power. In the design of magnetic products, the medical magnets must be placed in such a way as to form a closed electrical circuit to increase their power and to eliminate the south pole influence that is present at the edges of uni-pole magnets. There are more differences, but let's get back to what happened to Lucky.

Lucky is pitch black and weighs about 80 pounds—a perfect hostess to our dog, Little Dilly. She let Little Dilly lie in her spot by the pool and let him eat out of her dish and drink her water. Lucky loves medical magnets. Dolores put Lucky out one morning to let her run around a while. The humidity in Spring Hill is just like Florida, but the ground is like a desert. There are many poisonous snakes in the area, and Lucky loves to dig them up. Unfortunately, this time she was bitten by one. She barely made it home. Her head was swollen to twice its size, and she was near death. Chuck called the vet, and they said it was probably too late and that there was very little hope.

Bob had loaned Chuck a NeoMax for a painful muscle, and it worked. Chuck had studied magnetic therapy, so when Lucky got bitten, he knew exactly what to do. He knew that when a medical magnet is placed on the body, bodily fluids pass through the magnetic field. This rearranges the hydrogen molecule to change pH. Snake venom is very low in pH, or acidic. As the blood and bodily fluids pass through the magnetic field emitted from the NeoMax, the pH at that spot is immediately raised. Thus the pH is brought to normal at that spot and the venom is neutralized. Eventually all the blood circulates past the force fields emitted from the NeoMax and is neutralized.

Chuck went to work, and called home about two hours later. Lucky was going to be all right. She was up and moving around. He called home in another two hours and Lucky was eating and drinking, showing no sign that she had ever been bitten. As soon as we heard about Lucky, we called Dr. Philpott. He wasn't surprised. He commented, "Isn't it too bad everybody doesn't know about this? When you come to think about it, a NeoMax should be in every First Aid kit. Place it over any kind of insect or snake bite. The itch or pain will go away in a few minutes, or even seconds. Place it over a bump or a painful scrape, it helps heal and reduces or eliminates the pain."

Animals have aches and pains that we will never know about. I provide every animal I own with the appropriate magnetic device to make its life as enjoyable as possible while living. I follow the same strategy of helping my animals get out of pain or disease as I do myself. I use properly designed therapeutic magnets first, and then I consider other things. Usually the magnets work. Animals respond very favorably to magnetic therapy. The fact that their instincts cause them to want to stay close to the magnets says a lot. Some people hold instincts on the same level as the voice of God.

Chapter Seven

The Science of Physics

Magnetic Fields

A magnet looks like any other piece of metal. But when placed close to steel, it is easy to notice the difference. Magnets attract. A magnet is a power source that emits a force field. Its energy is organized at its poles.

The most common type of magnet is a bar magnet, especially those with one pole on each end.

If a string is tied to the middle of this type magnet and the magnet is allowed to swing by itself, the magnet's north pole will point to the earth's south pole. The reason is simple. Unlike poles attract.

If another bar magnet with the poles on its ends passes the south pole close to the suspended magnet's south pole, it will repel.

However, both poles attract steel and other materials that have magnetic properties. If a little piece of steel, such as a paper clip, is stroked over the pole of a magnet, the paper clip becomes a magnet too.

My Research

My research brought me to the NASA web site where I found this fascinating information. Magnetism is everywhere in outer space, but there is no magnetic iron. Sunspots are intensely magnetic, and they aren't even metal. They are, instead, gases like air only a lot hotter. Speaking of hot, the earth's magnetic fields generate from the intensely hot center of the earth, yet a bar magnet is completely cool.

All matter consists of electrically charged particles. Within each particle are molecules that have electrons. Each electron consists of light (negatively charged particles) moving around a positive nucleus. Whether a particle is negatively or positively charged depends on its electrons. If the particle has extra electrons, it is negatively charged, and if it is missing electrons, it is positively charged. Heat causes movement. Intense heat causes a dynamic thrashing around. In this bombarding of particles, electrons continuously get added to or lost to particles.

As far back as 1800, someone attached a metal wire to each end of a chemical battery and received a shock, quickly discovering the flow of electric current through wire. Electrons were hopping from atom to atom through out the wire. Thus, we could call electricity "electron-hopping."

A few years later Han Christian Oersted discovered that this "electron-hopping" caused a compass needle to move. Andre-Marie Ampere theorized that magnetism was associated with electrical current.

The NASA web site today offers this information: "Two parallel currents in the same direction attract each other. Two parallel currents in opposite directions repel each other." To create magnetism, take metal that possess magnetic properties such as iron, which contains chemical matter, and attach a long wire to one terminal. Coil it into circles at least a hundred times, and attach it to the other terminal. Place the metal inside coils. Thus, electricity is the source of magnetism.

The Lodestone

In the Greek city of Magnesia, people knew about strange and rare stones, which they called "lodestone." The Chinese, as well, knew about them, and they also had discovered that stroking the lodestone could make a magnet. If this new little magnet became suspended, it pointed either north or south. Thus, was the birth of the magnetic compass.

News soon spread to Europe, and when Columbus crossed the Atlantic, he used it as well. He knew how to determine true north from the stars. When he compared the newly created compass to the stars, he noticed a slight deviation, noticing, too, that this deviation changed as he moved across the ocean. Then William Gilbert figured out that the Earth is a giant magnet and its magnetic poles were not actually positioned at its geographic poles, which define the axis around which the Earth turns.

The Magnetosphere

The Earth's magnetic force field requires a very sensitive needle to detect. Farther out in space this field is even weaker. But beyond the Earth's dense atmosphere, forces play a bigger role. In this region, they dominate the environment. It is called the Earth Magnetosphere. It affects us very little. Fluctuations of the magnetic field are known as magnetic storms such as the "northern lights" that appear in the night skies visible from places such as Alaska and Norway. Satellites in space are affected much much more. Magnetic field lines and electromagnetic waves are two of the phenomena affecting our satellites and us to a lesser degree.

Magnetic Field Lines

Take a small jar of iron shavings and sprinkle them on a piece of paper. Take a magnet and place it under the paper. The iron shavings will form lines. These lines are called magnetic field lines and radiate from all magnets. Magnetic field lines of the Earth start near the south pole and curve around in space until they reach the north pole.

In the Earth magnetosphere, other currents change this neat, straight, direct pattern. On the side facing the sun, the magnetic field lines are compressed toward the Earth. On the other side, the night side, they are spiraling outward forming a long sort of tail something like that of a comet. In Faraday's day, it was thought that the only significance of these lines was to display the structure of this force field.

However, in space research, they have a much broader significance because electrons and ions tend to stay attached to them and become trapped under certain conditions. Because of the attraction, one can determine the direction from which they came as is possible to determine the direction of electric currents and certain radio waves.

Movement from one line to another is more difficult in space than on Earth. Scientists have created a map that shows the different regions of the magnetic field lines in the magnetosphere, how they are linked, and other important properties.

Electromagnetic Waves

While Faraday only thought of the space around a magnet as filled with magnetic field lines, his intuition that such space was modified led Scottish physicist James Clerk Maxwell to develop a mathematical model which merged magnetic field lines and electrical forces into one called electromagnetic waves. Electromagnetic waves became the cornerstone of the science of Physics. Maxwell's basic equation suggested that these waves were in motion and spreading with the speed of light. He guessed that light waves were a mix of certain variables of electromagnetic waves.

Heinrich Hertz produced the first light waves in a laboratory by electrical means in Germany. Today radio waves, microwaves, infra-red, visible light, ultra-violet, x-rays and gamma rays are all chunked into the category of electromagnetic waves.

Electromagnetic Radiation

The term radiation has been confused with other specific terms and has even become a thing in itself. The concept of radiation is very simple. It is merely a term to explain a force field traveling outward from a power source. It can be beneficial or good. For example, light radiates outward from the sun. Or, sound waves radiate from a person's vocal cords.

Electric current is defined as the movement of electrons through a wire. This current products two types of force fields. One is an alternating current (AC) electric field and the other is a magnetic field. Together they are called an electromagnetic field. The AC electric is the result of the strength of the charge and represents the force that electric charges exert on other charges. The magnetic fields result from the motion of the charge. This force can attract or repel. If you could see the magnetic force field, it would look like a donut circling the wire.

Most people can feel an electric field of about 20 kilovolts/meter as a tingling sensation on the skin. This kind of power can be found under high voltage power lines. Some people say they can feel AC magnetic force fields but most cannot.

Which came first, the AC electric field or the magnetic field? The electric field. AC electric current creates its own AC magnetic field. Then the AC magnetic field creates an AC electric current in a nearby conductor, thus the principle of induction. It is how we detect and measure AC electromagnetic fields. It is the principle by which a transformer raises or lowers voltage. This is the way a transformer works. When an AC electric current flowing through a coil of wire radiates an AC magnetic field, the adjacent coil of wire picks it up, then converts it back to AC electric current. To increase or decrease the amount of voltage, increase or decrease the number of coils.

The way transformers distribute electricity over a long distance is using very high voltage and then reducing and increasing the voltage at various points along the way. In an earlier chapter of this book, I explained the elements of a force field. I'll briefly do it again. A force field travels in a spiraling circle. The speed at which it travels is the number of times it can make a complete circle in one second. So, the speed is called "cycles per second" or can be referred to as "frequency." The direction in which it travels is either clockwise or counter-clockwise. This is the polarity. The size of the circle is the power usually measured in watts or in the case of permanent magnets the term "gauss" is used.

In the term "alternating current," have you ever wondered why it is called alternating? What alternates is the direction of the spin—or the polarity. This changing of direction is measured in hertz. In standard household current in the United States, the direction changes back and forth sixty times in one second. With straight magnetic current, it doesn't change direction at all and is referred to as direct current. A test instrument called an oscilloscope produces a view of this spiral that looks like a wave, hence the term "sine" wave is used. Sixty cycles per second is a very low frequency. Power plants generate this energy and it is "shipped" via lines to our homes, aided by capacitors. Energy, when it leaves the plant, is all energized and ready to go.

The problem is that is doesn't stay that way for long. Before it winds down completely, it flows through a device called a capacitor. Energy stays there until more arrives and builds and builds until it explodes outward and down the line to the next capacitor, each time losing a small amount of energy. Finally, the energy is directed to our home, and the voltage is slowed while traveling down my transformer so it won't over power our household electrical system.

The terms EMR (electromagnetic radiation) and EMF (electromagnetic frequency) are used interchangeably. EMR are all the waves in general and EMF is merely the fact that they are low frequency. Whether they are harmful or cancer causing is not defined in these terms. Starting with the low end of the scale and working upward in speed is: 1) ELE-- extremely low frequency, radio waves used by submarines for communication 2) VLF–very low frequency, which include microwaves, infrared (heat) waves, visible light, ultraviolet, s- rays and gamma rays. The rest are in the high frequency rating.

Science has come to define a type of radiation (force field) by its frequency because it determines its character. W-rays can strip electrons away from an atom to create an "ion." This is destructive to human tissue. Instantly a whole area of deformed cells are created. If the body has energy to spare, it will get right to business and repair them all. But if the body is sick or otherwise weakened and can spare no healing energy, then the cells just stay that way and reproduce in their defective state. This type of force field is called ionizing radiation because it tears up electrons, leaving them defective as ions. This is called cancer because the DNA is broken apart. (The DNA is the molecule that reproduces and makes our genes). When the frequency is low, it is said that the radiation is non-ionizing. This means it does not have the force or the ability to knock electrons away from or alter the molecular structure. However, it can still disrupt the entire molecule itself.

The good news is that this low frequency force field dissipates very quickly as it radiates outward from its source. It is almost ineffective by the time it travels just a couple of inches.

But, on the other hand, continuous exposure to them can be very harmful especially to a weakened body. Another consideration is the number of sources.

For example, I am sitting in my office at the computer. There are lights overhead. I have a printer off to the side. There is a refrigerator directly behind with a microwave oven on top of it.

The Gauss Meter

This instrument measures the strength of the magnetic field. It is made by winding a coil of thin wire several hundreds of turns. When this coil of wire is placed close to a magnetic field, the force field radiates through the coil.

This induces a current that is amplified by other circuitry and translated to a needle which moves to number on a scale. If a Gauss meter had about 40,000 turns, it would induce enough current to be read directly with a voltmeter.

Sometimes the term Tesla is used. A Tesla is 10,000 Gauss. The MRI is rated in Tesla.

Ancient Wisdom, Modern Use

Without magnetism, there would be no life. Life developed under the influence of the Earth's magnetic field. Magnetism plays a large role in health and disease. It all started when the

Greeks discovered lodestone. The metal staff of a shepherd stuck to it. Therapeutic benefits became known in a hit or miss fashion.

Wizards, witches, medicine men and other healers demonstrated its benefits. Magnetism became known as something magical. The Chinese culture took it to the next level in human benefit, but it was still thought of as mystical. More serious inquiry came over the years and Dr. Nakagowa wrote research papers--such as "Magnetic Deficiency Syndrome." This paper presented magnetism from a respected doctor's standpoint. It actually stated that a magnetic deficiency could cause just about anything you can think of. The paper specifically lists stress, mental disorder, headaches, arthritis, muscle pain, osteoporosis, chronic fatigue, allergies, insomnia, inflammation, circulatory problems, bowel disorders, and many degenerative problems.

They Are Just Force Fields

Electricity, magnetism, sound, and light are all the same. They are just force fields. Light is a combination of electric and magnetic fields. It changes very rapidly. You can turn off the lights at night in the winter, shuffle your feet across a dry carpet, then touch someone, and you will give that person a shock. The shock makes a sound and for a split second there is light. Take a balloon and rub it across a person's dry hair, then hold it a couple of inches above the person's head and watch hair stands stand on end. If you've done these experiments, you have just created force fields.

With each experiment, you create electricity, magnetism, sound and light. We already talked about how a bar magnet with the poles on opposite ends will align itself with the force fields of the earth. The magnet's north pole points to the south pole of the earth and its south pole points to the earth's north pole. This happens because the earth's south pole attracts the magnet's north pole and repels the magnet's south pole, while at the same time the Earth's north pole attracts the magnet's south pole and repels the magnet's north pole. So, you have four forces acting to align your suspended bar magnet.

James Clerk Maxwell studied force fields and made some landmark discoveries. He found that if electric charges are pushed or pulled, the changes in the speed of the charge creates magnetic fields. And vice versa. If the force fields of magnetism change, they create electricity. From this useful information, electric generators were created. Generators work by using the force fields of magnets to "push" electrical charges through wires. Thus, the magnetic fields are turned into electrical fields. This surge of electricity dies down and is built back up again with the magnets. It's like a wave in which the first part is magnetism and the second part is electricity. When one dies down, the other takes over.

Low Frequency Force Fields

Have you even listened to submarines talk to each other or to a base on land? It sounds like a monster is talking. This is because the frequency of the sound is very low. It has to be low because that is the only way it will pass through water. Recall the force field (a spiral) has only four elements that vary: 1) the speed in which it travels measured by the time it takes for a partical to travel around the circle in one second – called frequency or cycles per second, 2) the direction of the spin – either clockwise or counter-clockwise, referred to as the poles 3) the size of the circle, referred to as power, 4) the distance and intensity in which it can travel – determined by the size of the power source. The main variable (element) in a submarine's transmission is the low frequency. Because the frequency was so low, it couldn't travel through the air at all. It has to travel through water or earth. For a base station on earth to receive the frequency, it needs an antenna. We think of antennas as extending upward into the air and big ones high in the sky. But low frequency antennas are over a mile long and buried in the ground.

When this communication system was put in place, it was thought that because the frequency was so low they couldn't possibly cause significant biological changes. This reasoning was based upon the fact that low frequencies cannot break molecular bonds and generate only a minuscule amount of heat--not enough to heat body tissue.

However, low frequency or not, they still induce electric currents in a conductive medium. Because our bodies contain a large percentage of salt and water, we are a perfect conductive medium.

The way it affects life is not completely known by mainstream scientists. But I think I understand it. I believe it is a polarity issue. When the force field spins just one way, it is called "direct current" – DC. All harmful force fields are alternating energy patterns that spin one way then the other and back the first way again.

EMF'S

There are other low frequency force fields besides sound. We have named them EMF's. One theory of why they are harmful is that they disrupt the flow of calcium through the cells. Calcium acts as a messenger that penetrates the cell, conveying important information and triggering proteins to carry out cell functions.

Calcium also plays an important role in regulating certain body functions, such as muscle contractions, heartbeat, development of egg cells, and cell division. Since cancer growth depends on cell proliferation, these findings seem to explain why EMF sometimes behave like agents that promote, rather than initiate, cancerous growths.

Another theory is the resonance effect between EMF and the surfaces of the cells. This is like water pipes when they become noisy, shake, and begin to resonate. Usually a small flow of water does not cause this shaking. The flow is increased, and it gets louder. The flow is increased even more and the sound stops. In an oscilloscope, you can see a wave shape display. This is obtained by wiring this test instrument to an electrical source.

Changes in the source produce different shaped waves. Some scientists think certain wave shapes or wave shape changes are harmful.

ELF and VLF Radiation

There are two frequency ranges for magnetic fields which are commonly found around our homes and businesses: ELF (extremely low frequency) which radiates from a 60 Hz current, such as power lines, and VLF (very low frequency) which comes from the 15 kHz to 85 kHz scanning frequencies of TVs and cathode ray tube video displays.

The full ELF frequency range is between 0 Hz and 1,000 Hz, and the VLF range extends from 1,000 Hz (1 kHz) to 500,000 Hz (500 kHz). The problem with these frequency ranges is that they are alternating. They have to be alternating because direct current doesn't travel well for long distances.

Power Lines

In addition to the dangers of alternating frequencies is the power of the force field. An enormous amount of electricity is created at power-generating stations and sent across the country through wires that carry high voltages. These voltages can be 69,000, 100,000, 161,000, 230,000, 500,000, or even 765,000 volts. All power lines emit magnetic and electric fields. Combined with the fact that they are alternating, there is double trouble. The power emitted by a 500,000-volt transmission line can be as high as several hundred mG directly underneath the power line, and the field can still be measured more than a thousand feet away.

On top of it, all networks of secondary distribution lines crisscross most cities and towns, and these distribution lines have strong damaging force fields, even if you are 10-50 feet away. Interestingly, the amount of EMF coming from a high-power transmission line depends upon its particular configuration. This design was done for the efficient transmission of power. Back then they didn't realize there was any possibility of harm to biological life. Power companies know which power line configurations are best for reducing EMF, but most utilities feel that the evidence so far does not support costly changes in the way electricity is delivered.

To make the transmission of electricity safe requires compromises on everyone's part. For very little money, power companies can make a slight change in the most common line configuration called a "vertical double-circuit." This is a set of three cables attached one on top of the other, to each side of the transmission tower. The three cables comprise the three phases that are deliberately set out of phase with each other.

Time Out

Did I lose you in the technical talk? Think of the spiral from the side. You can see a wave. It peaks up and down. If all three cables peaked at the same time, they would be in phase. But they all peak at slightly different times to make the out of phase. They are labeled A-B-C. In 1989, Booneville Power Administration changed the configuration to C-B-A. It cut down the EMF immediately.

The compromise came in because there was a buzzing and snapping noise in nearby televisions and radios that caused interference. Entertainment or health--that is the question.

It is also possible to position the three lines side by side in a flat configuration called a "delta" configuration. This cancels the harmful EMFs but makes it more dangerous for the maintenance workers and degrades the performance during lightning.

Burying the cable reduces EMF but the buried cable still has to be configured properly. If it is not, the EMF can radiate from the ground. The person can't see it, doesn't know it, and is hurt and doesn't know why, especially if the underground service is a single-phase wire. In this case, it is more harmful than overhead wires because the person is closer to it.

Most popular wire configurations that reduce EMF are less efficient and, therefore, cost more. But power companies are researching and developing new ways.

In one new design, they are putting the wires in pipes filled with oil that cools the cable. They found that EMF can be reduced even further by grounding the cables in a special way.

Substation

Industrial-looking complexes of equipment with chain-linked fences around them are of little interest to most of us. Children ask their parents what is that--but the parents rarely know. We all have better things to do than to learn about someone else's job. It is all we can do to function in this complex world and do our own. Until there is a good reason to even wonder about substations we just ignore them and continue to live our lives.

However, the following account provides the reason we need to not only learn about substations but also shows why we need to get involved in the running of them. Meadow Street, in the little town of Guildford, CT, was written about in the

New Yorker on July 9, 1990. The unusual thing about this street was the incidence of cancer per number of residences living on the street. In a 20-year period there were four brain tumors, one eye tumor, one ovarian tumor, and one bone tumor for a total of seven. All these people with cancer lived close to the substation.

A substation is an assemblage of circuit breakers, disconnecting switches, and transformers designed to change and regulate the voltage of electricity. Primary distribution lines, carrying high voltages typically of 115,000 volts to 230,000 volts, bring the current from the power plant to the substation, where the transformers reduce it to lower voltages, typically 4,000 to 13,800 volts.

The transformers give off magnetic fields because they depend upon magnetic fields to operate. My question: What kind of magnetic fields?

The answer is it probably doesn't matter because the power is so high anyway. My thinking is that perhaps if they make a mere polarity change, they may be able to reduce the damage or may even stop it all together. To further compound the problem, the incoming and outgoing currents at a substation are generally unbalanced, and high magnetic fields from substations have been blamed for causing cancer clusters among nearby residents. (Paul Brodeur called this "cancer clusters.") Meadow Street only had nine houses on it, making this very unlikely to be normal. And right next to the substation was a 115,000 volt high-current distribution line which fed the current to the substation. The measurements at the fence ranged from 20mG to several hundred mG.

Transformers

Part of the distribution system that enables the delivery of electricity to each home is the transformer. It looks like a metal trashcan. The purpose of this is to "transform" the power from the high power used to transport it to the lower power so the home can use it. The voltage could be as high as 14,000. Even when the service is underground, they still need transformers and wires feeding into it, and these can be extremely high voltage. But the good thing is that the field quickly diminishes as the distance from it increases. So unless you must walk very close to it, there shouldn't be much of a problem. On the other hand, with something so potentially dangerous, it wouldn't hurt to ask some questions of the utility company or test the fields yourself.

Wiring Inside Your Home

You can't tell by looking at a wire if there is current flowing through it or not. So, it's always a good rule of thumb to never touch wires at all. Even if you know the wire is disconnected, there still could be a stray field around the wire and exposure for several hours on a regular basis could cause cancer.

Another reason not to touch or be in contact with wires is because it is possible the wiring is not installed correctly somewhere else in the house. Household current comes through two hot wires and one neutral wire called a ground. For appliances that require 240 service, the two "hots" are put together. Other things in the home that require 120 only require one "hot." Modern homes have electrical outlets with three holes--two rectangles and a smaller half-round hole at the bottom. The rectangle on the right is smaller, and this is for the hot wire. The rectangle on the left is larger, and this is for the neutral wire. The small half-round hold at the bottom is for the ground.

While keeping tabs on the utility company and making sure you are not in jeopardy of the high powered fields is important, something far more important and much, much easier to control is your own household wiring. Years ago it was a standard practice to connect the ground wire to a water pipe. Let's examine this and figure out why it is or why it is not a good practice. Let's consider the circuitry of a refrigerator as an example.

Power is generated in a plant, travels to your home, and enters at the panel box. From there it goes through fuses or circuit breakers that fly open to shoot off the flow of current if there is a surge or a spike of power. These fuses or circuit breakers save our appliances from taking these kinds of blows that could burn up the appliances--but does no harm at all to a breaker. However, the spikes and surges destroy a 25 cent fuse rather than a several hundred-dollar appliance.

The power then leaves the panel box and travels to the refrigerator. The wires take it to the motor, which starts to turn as the power comes on. A blower runs, a compressor starts to cool the air, and so on. Electricity makes its rounds in the refrigerator's circuitry and then flows back to the panel box in a closed loop. This closed loop cancels out any stray fields making sure all the current gets used and none is wasted. Over time, the wires dry out, are heated and cooled, could be stepped on, animals could chew on them--for whatever reason they could become frayed. A frayed wire creates an additional demand on current for no reason. To handle this excessive current, the ground wire is attached to the refrigerator's frame. This means that any stray or excessive current will flow into the refrigerator's frame instead of the person.

If this neutral wire is attached to the plumbing instead of running back to the panel box, it could create a significant and harmful force field. Why? Because water is a good conductor of electricity. And water pipes sometimes sweat and come in direct contact with the home's electricity. Tracing the flow of the electric current from the panel box to the refrigerator, after the electric current powers the refrigerator, it will run to the neutral and, if wired incorrectly, through the plumbing where it is grounded. Since it is no longer paired with the hot wire, the magnetic field will not cancel out. Instead, there will be a magnetic field around the hot wire that is connected to the refrigerator and another field may surround all your plumbing. Just one incorrectly grounded appliance can send electricity through all your water pipes and create a magnetic field throughout your entire house!

This practice "provides an alternate path for the [neutral return] current to flow from your house back to the distribution system," says Gary Johnson, an executive at a General Electric facility doing EMF research for the Electric Power Research Institute. As a result, an imbalance is created which reduces the canceling effect of the neutral's field on the hot conductor. This little-known fact can be an eye opener for explaining mysterious EMF in some homes.

According to Johnson, you could create fields in your neighbor's house when you switch your appliances on and off, and your neighbor could create them in your house, too. This phenomenon can also account for fields outside of the home and in overhead distribution lines.

Quoting from the NASA web site: Changing the plumbing from metal to plastic is not a proper solution because electric current is not supposed to flow through the plumbing. The only solution is to rewire correctly, with all hot and neutral wires paired closely together and without any current flowing through the ground wire or through plumbing. Another source of EMF comes from the power line where it enters your home. The area of your home near this feeder line will have a reading, even if the rest of the house is properly wired.

If your supply line enters your home with an overhead wire, as opposed to underground, you may want to avoid using a corner of your home, or part of a room, for any prolonged period of time. To test your home for magnetic fields, walk through your home with an ELF Gauss meter. If the reading is generally below 1.0 mG except near appliances, your home is wired correctly. If you find extensive zones of higher readings, you need to first determine if the EMF is coming from your own wiring or from a source outside your home. To start, walk outside and see what the readings are around your home. Then turn off your electricity at your panel box and check inside your home. The results will tell you if you need to go further and check your wiring.

If you find high readings, it is time to call an electrician. First, have him or her verify your findings by isolating one circuit at a time. The electrician can test for the presence of unwanted ground currents with a clamp-on ammeter attached to your plumbing. It should read zero. However, the gauss meter is more sensitive and doesn't require you to open your plumbing. Hopefully you will find one incorrectly wired circuit but there is always a possibility that your entire house needs re-wiring.

Automatic icemakers in refrigerators and in-sink disposal units are often the source of unwanted EMF since copper piping to your plumbing usually connects these devices. It is important that these devices be wired so that no current flows through the ground.

Computer Terminals

ELF (Extra Low Frequency) ranging from 50 kilo Hertz to 80 kilo Hertz, and VLF (Very Low Frequency) ranging from 15 kilo Hertz to 85 kilo Hertz electromagnetic radiation from CRT-style screens is presently being considered dangerous. Why? Because this is all south pole, harmful energy, and second, the healthy human body resonates at 70 Mega Hertz. ELF radiation comes from the vertical deflection coils, and VLF radiation results from the horizontal deflection coils. CRT-style VDTs also have a power transformer that creates a 60 Hz field, and a fly back transformer, which steps up the CRT's voltage to tens of thousands of volts and emits VLF electromagnetic radiation. The levels of EMF emitted by a VDT can be quite high, but they dissipate exponentially with distance. That's why it is important to sit back at least an arm's length from the front of the screen.

Measurements taken from a 13-inch color screen was used for this test. It showed 37 mG of ELF at 6 inches, 12.6 mG at 12 inches and 4.5 mG at 20 inches. The VLF field (which contains several hundred times more energy than an ELF field at the same mG reading) is 6.3 mG at 6 inches, 2.0 mG at 12 inches, and .66 mG at 20 inches. At 6 to 7 feet the ELF level drops to background, but the VLF level is still measurable 10 feet away.

Because the EMF comes from the internal components, the EMF levels on the back and sides of a VDT are higher than in front, often by a factor of 2. This means you must distance yourself further away from the back and sides of a VDT (at least 3 to 4 feet, respectively) in order to achieve the same level of exposure. Smaller VDTs are not necessarily better, either. A 12-inch VDT might well generate a stronger magnetic field than a 19-inch one, because the field's strength depends more on the internal design of the deflection coils and electronic components than on the screen size. Monochrome displays typically produce 1/2 to 1/5 the levels of EMF than color displays, although this is not always the case. For example, a 9-inch display emitted a field of .30 mG of VLF at 20 inches in front of the screen. The electric components of a VDT consist of electrostatic potential and alternating electric fields at ELF, VLF, and radio frequencies. The electrostatic potential results from a build-up of an electric charge on the surface of the screen. Its effect is similar to what most of us experience when we get a static shock by walking across a carpet and touching a metal object in a dry environment. This static may attract dust on your screen and cause eye irritation. On some occasions, skin irritations have been reported, although this is infrequent and the cause has not been proven.

Fortunately, no long-term or serious health effects have been attributed to the electrostatic or alternating electric fields. However, incorporating a grounded conductive layer into an anti-glare shield can easily block the electric fields. On the other hand, ELF and VLF magnetic radiation is not easy to block.

Low-frequency magnetic fields can easily travel through layers of solid aluminum, copper or steel with little reduction in strength. Furthermore, unlike an electric field that travels in a straight line, a magnetic field loops outward in curves, forming an irregular, rounded envelope of energy.

Adding to the problem is the source of the EMF, which is not the front of the screen but the deflection coils, fly back transformer, and power supply inside the VDT. The EMF travels up and over the top of the screen, around the sides, and underneath in all directions. "Screen savers" designed to blank out the screen after a short period of inactivity are useful to prevent "burn in" or damage to the VDT's phosphor coating from constant use, but even if the image is blank, the components which generate ELF and VLF emissions are still active. Similarly, dimming the display will do nothing to reduce the fields. Shields placed in front of a VDT's screen do not block ELF magnetic fields. They do block electric fields, but the ELF magnetic field is the main concern.

When you hear the term, "radiation" you think that lead shielding is a solution. It isn't. Unlike X-rays, ELF and VLF magnetic fields can penetrate right through lead. One shielding method, which has shown partial success, is to install a Mu metal barrier around the deflection coils and fly back transformer inside the cabinet of the VDT. Mu metal is an alloy of nickel, iron, and various other trace metals, which is magnetically permeable, meaning that it is a good conductor of magnetic lines of force. The percentage of each element in the Mu metal affects its performance, as does the thickness and the method of manufacture. While Mu metal can reduce magnetic radiation if installed properly, it cannot block all the radiation in the same way that lead blocks out X-rays.

Mu metal is not recommended as a do-it-yourself solution for several reasons. The configuration and placement of the Mu metal will vary with each different model of VDT, sometimes requiring many hours of experimentation to determine the optimum configuration, and frequently its use may cause distortion in the image, which may mean the hiring of a service technician to adjust. Moreover, because the Mu metal redirects the magnetic fields, it is possible to actually increase fields, rather than reduce them. And last but not least, CRT-style VDTs can provide a dangerous electric shock if you don't know what not to touch, since the tube stores up thousands of volts, even when it is not plugged into the wall. In short, using Mu metal is an art rather than a science. In response to users' concerns, many display manufacturers have modified their VDTs to produce lower levels of magnetic radiation. Some low radiation models use a compensating coil adjacent to the deflection coils to create an opposite magnetic field. When the two opposing fields meet, most of the radiation is canceled out. Low radiation displays may also incorporate extra shielding around the yoke and fly back transformer.

What you don't know can hurt you. This is great cause for health concerns. IBM has obtained a patent on a device which reduces VDT radiation, and the company is using this technology to reduce the EMF coming from its displays. Other studies concerning the effects of EMF on embryos show reason for concern. According to Dr. Ezra Berman of the Environmental Protection Agency, "the Henhouse Study [of chicken embryos exposed to low-frequency magnetic fields] performed in four countries has contributed a database implicating an association of EMF with an increase of abnormalities in chick embryos."

Expert Louis Slesin, publisher of *VDT News*, says, "The new results should help convince skeptics that magnetic fields can be biologically active at very low levels."

However, pregnant women and their unborn fetuses are not the only ones at risk. CRT-style VDTs can emit levels of ELF magnetic radiation, which is far higher than 2 to 3 mG (the level associated with higher risks of brain tumors, leukemia and other cancers). A link between VDT use and cancer has not been established, but this does not mean there is no danger. Consider the fact that the vast majority of VDT operators in the U.S. are women and that the incidence of female breast cancer has been rising steadily along with VDT use.

Breast cancer now accounts for 29 percent of all cancers among women, and astounding 1 out of 9 women will contract it. Remember that power lines have been around for one hundred years, and the cancer link is just now being established. It took over forty years of research to conclusively establish the dangers of smoking. VDTs have only been widely used for the past twenty years. Purchase your low-radiation VDT from a reputable company, or bring along a Gauss meter and buy the display with the lowest emission levels.

Lap Top Computers

Laptop computers are made of liquid crystal displays (LCDs). Because this screen is backlit or side lit with fluorescent light, they also emit dangerous, south pole fields in the VLF and ELF range. The good news is the fields aren't as powerful as a regular computer screen. The bad news is that they could be just as harmful because a person can hold them on their lap, which is closer--and the closer the more harmful.

There are also electro luminescent displays, which emit similar levels of EMF as LCDs, and gas plasma monitors have a high electric and magnetic fields within a few inches of the display, but these fields drop off rapidly.

Televisions

Televisions emit the same assortment of radiation as computer displays, since both devices incorporate a cathode ray tube (CRT). Fortunately, a viewer doesn't have to sit right next to a television set to see the image.

Sitting ten feet away from a 19-inch television distances the viewer from any measurable ELF or VLF fields. Some televisions, though, are particularly strong, so it makes sense to test your television with both an ELF and VLF Gauss meter

A Gauss meter is also useful when buying a television, since sets can vary quite a bit from one another. Many appliances generate AC electric and AC magnetic fields even when they are turned off. For example, televisions with remote controls still have current flowing when not in use, and this current generates EMF although it is less than when the set is in use. Radios, too, may produce EMF even when turned off. If you need to watch television in a confined space, you should consider purchasing a small LCD television set.

They have quite a strong electric field at one inch, but at the distance of one foot, both the electric and magnetic fields are negligible.

Electric Blankets

Electric blankets create an AC magnetic field that penetrates about six or seven inches into the body. Thus it is not surprising that an epidemiological study has linked electric blankets with miscarriages and childhood leukemia

The major U.S. electric blanket manufacturers--Fieldcrest, Casco-Belton and Northern Electric (Sunbeam)--have come out with "zero magnetic field" blankets. In one design the wires are laid out in pairs so that the magnetic fields are balanced. Another design uses DC electricity, which doesn't emit pulsed EMF.

Although these models reduce or eliminate magnetic fields, the blanket may still produce electric fields, even when turned off. This is because current does not have to be flowing for an electric field to exist. If the on/off switch cuts the neutral wire instead of the hot wire, the user would then be subjected to the electric field coming from the hot wire in the blanket.

That's why it is best to use an electric blanket only to warm your bed before you get in it. Once you're in bed, the blanket should be unplugged to be absolutely safe. His advice is especially valid for children and pregnant women.

Electric Clocks

A dial-face (analog) electric clock has a very high AC magnetic field, as much as 5 to 10 mG up to two feet away. If you are using a bedside plug-in dial-face alarm clock, it should not be placed near your head

Fluorescent Lights

Fluorescent lights have replaced incandescent ones in most offices and schools. Fluorescent lights are cooler, last longer, and consume less electricity, so they are more economical to use. A fluorescent bulb has no filament but instead is coated on the inside with a fluorescent material called a phosphor. The bulb is also filled with argon gas and mercury vapor, and a transformer (called a ballast) is used to increase the voltage to the electrodes on each end of the bulb.

The high voltage excites electrons in the gas, which give off ultraviolet light, which strikes the phosphor coating on the bulb emitting visible light, which passes through the glass. Fluorescent lights produce much more EMF than incandescent bulbs: at a distance of two inches from an incandescent bulb, the ELF field is .3 mG, and at six inches it is barely measurable.

On the other hand, a typical fluorescent lamp of the type commonly found in office ceilings can have a reading of 160 to 200 mG one inch away. At six inches, the reading drops to 45 mG, at twelve inches the reading is 14 mG, at twenty-four inches the level is 1.7 mG, and at thirty inches the level is close to background. Thus, rooms with low ceilings and fluorescent lights may have readings above 2 mG at head level.

In multi-story schools with fluorescent lights, although young children may be far enough away from the ceiling fixtures, they may still be exposed to EMF from the lights on the floor below.

Microwave Ovens

Microwave ovens are interesting because they emit two types of radiation--microwave and ELF. The microwave radiation, which is very high in frequency (in the billion Hertz range), is produced by an element called a magnetron.

Microwaves make water molecules vibrate, and it is this vibration that creates the heating process. Not surprisingly, stray microwaves can cause serious health problems by heating body tissue.

Telephones

Telephones can emit surprisingly strong EMF, especially from the handset. This is a problem because we hold phones so close to our heads. Measuring different telephones before you buy is important because the field strength can vary a great deal in just a matter of inches. Place a Gauss meter right against the earpiece and the mouthpiece.

There are several telephone handsets in the market with no measurable fields, while others emit a relatively strong field that travels several inches. That's the same distance from your ear to your brain! As with most small appliances, the casing of the telephone has a magnetic field that extends one or two feet. Because of this, it is a good practice to position the phone as far as possible from the user.

Electric Razors and Hair Dryers

An electric razor, which plugs into the wall, produces an extremely high-strength AC magnetic field, as high as 200 to 400 mG one-half inch away from the cutting edge. This seems alarming, but we don't know if this is worse (or better) than exposure to a 2 to 3 mG field (the level linked to increased risk of cancer). If exposure to such high fields is a problem, the duration of the exposure (the dose-rate concept) might mitigate the effects.

To understand the dose-rate concept, consider that we can zip a finger through the flame of a match without burning ourselves. This is evidence that short-term exposure to certain harmful influences can produce dramatically different results than longer exposure. If the dose-rate concept applies to EMF (and we don't know if it does), since an electric razor is used only a few minutes each day, it is probably safe. Keep in mind, however, that the data on short-term exposure to high-strength fields is incomplete, and that the use of non-electric razor blades will eliminate all EMF risks.

Evidence—EMF's Are Unhealthy

One of the earliest studies on the human health effects of EMF was conducted in the greater Denver, Colorado area by epidemiologist Nancy Wertheimer and physicist Ed Leeper. Using data on children who had died before age nineteen of cancer between 1950 and 1979, this study found significant excess risks among children who resided in homes close to heavy-duty distribution lines.

In 1982, the *New England Journal of Medicine* published a letter from Dr. Samuel Milham, Jr. describing his study of leukemia deaths in Washington State. His comprehensive study, which examined the data for 438,000 deaths occurring between 1950 and 1979, found that leukemia deaths were elevated in 10 out of 11 occupations involving exposure to EMF.

In 1988, epidemiologist Dr. David Savitz set out to disprove the results of the earlier Denver study using a different group of children. Instead, his findings were nearly identical with the first study indicating elevated risk for all cancers among children living in homes near power lines with magnetic fields at or above 2 milliGauss (mG).

Perhaps the most publicized study was conducted in 1988 by the Kaiser Permanente HMO in Oakland, California, one of the largest health care facilities in the country. Kaiser's researchers tracked 1,583 pregnancies to discover if pregnant women had been affected by the widespread use of a spray that had been used to kill med flies.

No problem was found with the spraying, but the researchers were surprised to find a statistically significant 73% increase in miscarriages in working women using CRT-style VDTs (cathode ray tube video display terminals), compared to other working women. The study also found an increase in birth defects, although the result was not statistically significant due to the sample size.

A Johns Hopkins study showed that the incidence of leukemia among telephone cable workers was seven times greater than among other telephone company employees.

A subsequent study of 1.5 million past and present employees of AT&T found that men working as cable splicers and central office technicians had 1.7 times the risk of dying from leukemia than men working at jobs with less exposure to EMF. This is startling, considering that the field these men are exposed to is, on the average, relatively low (4.3 milliGauss.)

Studies of cells and laboratory animals exposed to EMF show biological effects, including changes in levels of neurotransmitters--the chemicals which send signals between nerves--changes in levels of calcium found inside or on the surface of cells, embryo abnormalities in chickens, mice and pigs, malignant lymphomas in mice exposed to very high-intensity EMF, slowing of repetitive learning and reduced testicle weight in rats, changes in brain chemistry, heightened stress, and changes in the rate of growth and cell division of some cells.

The latter effects have implications for the offspring of pregnant women and growing children. In some experiments, human cancer cells exposed to EMF exhibit increased resistance to attack by the body's cancer-fighting white blood cells and the body's immune system. Furthermore, a drop in the levels of melatonin has been reported in people sleeping with electric blankets. Melatonin is a hormone that controls the monthly female cycle and inhibits the growth of certain cancers.

Prudent Avoidance

So what do you do? Electricity makes our lives easier. Electricity makes our lives less healthy and shorter. Unless we live in a cave and hardly ever see anyone we are going to be exposed to the dangers of electricity.

Electricity is an inseparable part of our modern day society. This means that electromagnetic radiation will continue to be all around us for the foreseeable future.

First

- Measure your environment with a Gauss meter and avoid areas where the field is above 1 mG. Measure the fields both inside and outside your home, and don't let your children play near power lines, transformers, and microwave towers.

- Measure the magnetic fields from appliances, both when they are operating and when they are turned off. Magnetic fields are created only when current is flowing, but some appliances (such as TVs) draw current even when switched off.

- Don't sleep under an electric blanket or on a waterbed. If you want to warm your bed before going to sleep, when you're ready to get under the cover, unplug the electric blank. Don't just turn it off. Even though there is no magnetic field when the blanket is off, there may still be a high electric field.

- Don't sit too close to your television set. Stay at least six feet, but keep in mind that EMF from some sets can be measured as far as ten feet or more. An ELF and VLF Gauss meter can help you decide where to sit.

- Keep at least an arm's length away from the screen,

and remember that at this distance, you'll be within the magnetic field. Computer monitors vary in the strength of the magnetic fields they emit, so check yours with an ELF and VLF meter.

- Rearrange your office work area so that you and your co-workers are not exposed to EMF from the sides and backs of each other's VDTs.

- Turn off your VDT when you are not using it.

- Consider purchasing a low-radiation VDT, which contains an active compensating coil, or a zero-radiation display based on shielded LCD technology.

- Don't stand close to your microwave oven when in use. Even if your microwave oven is not leaking microwaves, it will still give off strong ELF magnetic fields.

- Move your electric clock away from your pillow—several feet away should be sufficient. Better yet, buy a battery-powered digital clock.

- Keep other electric appliances away from your pillow, too. Telephones and answering machines generate EMF.

- Eliminate dimmers and three-way switches; they create highfields.

- Eliminate wires running under your bed.

- Be wary of cordless appliances such as electric tooth brushes that use magnetic induction to charge the battery. Such devices deliberately create a large magnetic field.

- Remember that EMF passes right through walls, so check out what is on the other side. It could be a cordless electric toothbrush, or a television set, or a clock-thermostat radiating EMF into your bedroom.

Some Answers—Magnets to the Rescue

Nineteen patients in a well-designed scientific study published in the *American Journal of Pain Management* wore magnetic insoles 24 hours a day except while showering. They then rated their pain twice a day for 4 months.

The trick was making sure the pain relief was really due to the magnets. Test subjects inserted magnetic insoles into their shoes.

"I created a design to have the patient test one foot as a control against a real magnet in the other foot, and then after one month, switch them so in the other month they would have a magnet in the opposite foot and a sham magnet or a sham device on the other foot, so they would not know which ones they were," Dr. Weintraub explained.

Both the foot with the fake and the real magnet got some pain relief but when they were switched to real magnets, 90 percent of the diabetics got significantly better from their neuropathy. Castner said, "Since the magnetic chips, it's ironic how I don't —I still have numbness, but it's decreased."

—*National Institute of Neurological Disorders and Stroke: Peripheral Neuropathy Dr. Max Gomez*

Summary of 12-Month, Clinical Test of Magnetic Mattress Pads

The mattress pads used in this study were typical full-size pads containing 124 permanent ferrite magnets with magnetic field strengths of 750-950 gauss each. The pads themselves were made of two sheets of felt with the magnets sandwiched between them. The felt sheets were then wrapped in a cloth cover. The total number of subjects in this double-blind clinical experiment was 431 (216 male, 215 female). 375 subjects were given magnetic pads, 56 were given non-magnetic pads. None of the 431 subjects knew which pad they were sleeping on. Subjects selected for the experiment were those with chief complaints related to neck and shoulder pain, back and lower back pain, back pain (general), lower limb pain, insomnia and fatigue. To determine the presence of any side effects, blood pressure, hemoglobin, number of erythrocytes and number of leucocytes were examined before and after the use of the mattress pads. Besides blood sedimentation, and TP, COL, ALT, GOT, GPT, Na, and K were also examined, as were functions of the kidneys, liver, pancreas, and the entire circulatory system. Out of 375 total subjects with symptoms, 301 (80.27 percent) reported positive results. 74 cases (19.73 percent) reported no results

The percentage of subjects who realized the effect of the magnetic mattress pad within 3 days: neck and shoulder pain 46.9 percent, back and lower back pain 50 percent, back pain (general) 38.7 percent, lower limb pain 54.4 percent, insomnia 64.3 percent, and fatigue 57.8 percent.

Out of 375 total subjects who slept on magnetic mattress pads, 200(53.3 percent) realized the effects within three days. Over 70 percent realized the effects within five days.

Testing for side effects was conducted at the conclusion of the experiment. Symptoms such as tinnitus, headache, hearing problems, visual disturbances, vertigo, palpitation, perceptive abnormality, motor disturbance, fever, digestive disturbance, cutaneous symptoms and other clinical symptoms to suggest any side effects were found to be totally absent.

Extensive testing was also done before and after the experiment to check functions of the kidney, liver, pancreas, blood pressure, and circulatory system. No clinical symptoms were found to indicate any side effects whatsoever.

Dr. Shimodaira's conclusion of this year-long study conducted in three of Japan's foremost hospitals: "The magnetized health mattress (pad) is proved to be effective on neck and shoulder pain, back and lower back pain, back pain, lower limb pain, insomnia and fatigue, and to have no side effects."

Magnets — Universal Cure All?

Dr. Kazuo Shimodaira of the Tokyo Communications Hospital and Kouseikai Suzuki Hospital suggests that in the search for a universal cure-all, none fits the description nearly as well as magnetic energy therapy. The application of magnets has given a proven pain relief in seven out of ten users--as good or better than "orthodox" medicine. Magnetotherapy is far less expensive and has no dangerous side effects often seen with prescription drugs; however, proper advice and care should be taken when using strong or large magnets about the head. Treatment with magnets is not addictive and does not interfere with other therapies but should not be used if a pacemaker or defibrillator is worn.

Researchers have stated that magnetic field therapy re-balances altered metabolic functions that cause pain such as edema, excess acid in the tissues, and lack of oxygen in the cells, thereby initiating tissue healing and pain relief.

Skin calcification, the cause of skin aging and wrinkles, disappears while joint mobility increases and muscles become more flexible. Digestion and elimination improve, prostates shrink, and kidneys eliminate body wastes more effectively. Mental function increases, energy levels increase, and sleep is better.

Tests have shown that organisms placed under a magnetic field live longer. Because it potentates the body's free radical scavenger and antioxidant system, magnetic therapy is reported to be valuable in counteracting degenerative processes that cause heart and circulatory diseases, arthritis and auto-immune illness, and neuro-degenerative and allergic afflictions.

Natural Pain Relief, According to Ken Wiancko, MD
Drinking magnetized water is said to impart many similar benefits. Wearing back, neck or joint supports with permanent magnets imbedded in the material often relieves painful conditions. Treatment of discomfort from strains and arthritis with low-frequency pulsating magnetic fields created by tiny portable generators may be as effective as larger ultrasound units. Stress causes hundreds of diseases; using magnets day or night can reduce it. Sleeping on magnetic mattress pads can improve the quality of sleep and eliminate morning stiffness. Nighttime magnetic field therapy has a calming and sleep-inducing effect of the brain and body due to stimulating production of the hormone melatonin.

Melatonin is anti-stressful, anti-aging and anti-infectious. Magnetic therapy may often by used as a first line of treatment for pain and to promote healing.

This is not to suggest that there is no place for standard prescription drugs, but that many distressing conditions yield to magnets. If magnets don't help, it's important that you visit your doctor.

How Magnetism Works by Dr. H.L. Bansel
Biomagnetism works in the human body through the circulatory, nervous, and endocrine systems. Magnetism is continuously penetrating every known particle, right down to the atom. Its ordering effect on living systems arises from the fact that magnetism is a blueprint of life itself. All known energies have as a base this electromagnetic field, and the latest research indicates that magnetism has a very significant biological effect on human beings. Dr. H.L. Bansel points out that magnetism increases the electrical conductivity of the

blood. A weak current runs through it, increasing the quantity of ions, and the newly ionized blood circulating throughout the body can significantly contribute to the efficiency of the blood flow as well as having a stabilizing effect on both high and low blood pressure. Blood contains ferrous hemoglobin (iron) that functions as a carrier of oxygen and carbon dioxide. As the blood circulates in the lungs, fully magnetized ferrous hemoglobin is able to transport more oxygen to cell tissue as well as taking more carbon dioxide waste from the cells back to the lungs for removal. This means more energy and less fatigue as tissue cells and internal organs stay substantially healthier. In addition, therapeutic magnets work to regulate and normalize hormone secretion in the glands. It is currently believed that the increased electrical current being produced forms like a net around the glands and secretory duct.

An extra concentration of oxygen stimulates production while the electrical net regulates optimum secretion. As a result, conditions caused by a lack of hormone secretion or a hormone imbalance are affected through normalizing the hormone functions within the body.

Hormones play a very important role in rejuvenation and in general energy levels while proper circulation ensures that the hormone level is evenly distributed to all parts of the body. When magnetic flux passes through tissue, a secondary current is created around the flux lines in the tissue cells. This function of the cell becomes strengthened as the cell metabolism responds to the bioelectrical currents initiated by the magnetic flux.

This current induces muscle spasms to reduce, and the activated cell metabolism lowers inflammation in the tissue. The increase of cellular metabolism aids in the regeneration as well as in new cell growth. The negative pole energies of magnetism interfere with the nerve cells' ability to send pain impulses to the brain for the pain to be registered. Blood cells have potassium in their centers, which has a positive bioelectric charge. The nerve cell differs in an opposite way. During a pain response, the outside switches to potassium with a positive bioelectric charge. Through attraction, the negative pole charge of a magnet creates a "blend off" of the potassium's positive bioelectric as the natural flow of current is toward the negative pole.

Magnets stimulate blood circulation and building new cells to rejuvenate the tissues of the body. The biomagnetic effect on iron hemoglobin activates movement, thereby, activating circulation in a remarkable way.

Ineffective and weakened blood cells are appropriately strengthened, and more fresh vital blood is pumped into the system. With the respiratory exchange improved and cellular metabolism activated to increase vitality, prevention and cure of disease become a natural conclusion.

In summary, when a magnet is applied to the human body, magnetic waves pass through the tissues and secondary currents are induced. When these currents clash with magnetic waves, they produce impacting heats on the electrons in the body cells. The impacting waves are very effective to reduce pains and swellings in the muscles.

Movement of hemoglobin in blood vessels is accelerated while calcium and cholesterol deposits in blood are decreased. Even the other unwanted materials adhered to the inner side of blood vessels, which provoke high blood pressure, are decreased and made to vanish; the blood is cleansed and circulation is increased. The activity of the heart eases and pain disappears.

Functions of autonomic nerves are normalized so that the internal organs controlled by them regain their proper function.Secretion of hormones is promoted with the result that the skin gains luster, youth is preserved, and all the ailments due to the lack of hormone secretion are relieved and cured.

Blood and lymph circulation is activated and, therefore, all nutrients are easily and efficiently carried to every cell of the body. This helps in promoting general metabolism. Magnetic waves penetrate the skin, fatty tissues and bones, invigorating the organs. The result is greatly enhanced resistance to disease. The magnetic flux promotes health and provides energy by eliminating disorders in and stimulating the functions of the various systems of the body, namely the circulatory, nervous, respiratory, digestive, and urinary.

Magnetic treatment works by reforming, reviving and promoting the growth of cells, rejuvenating the tissues of the body, strengthening the decayed and inactive corpuscles, and increasing the number of new, sound corpuscles.

Magnets have exceptional curative effects on certain complaints like toothache, stiffness of shoulders and other joints, pains and swellings, cervical sponcylitis, eczema, asthma, as well as on chilblains, injuries, and wounds. The self-curative faculty (Homeostasis) of the body is improved and strengthened which ensures all the benefits mentioned above. One feels in full vigor and can walk and work more and more without feeling tired.

The magnetic treatment has the effect of energizing all the systems of the body, an effect that remains for several hours after each sitting with the magnets.

How Magnets Work by William Pawluk, M.D.

Magnets stimulate the acupuncture points and meridians. In this way, they can be used for all kinds of problems, especially for pain, fibromyalgia, and strains. They work on red blood cells because they contain iron.

Dr. Pawluk's nurse had a bad bruise on her knee from a ski injury and he placed a round Bulls-eye magnet directly over the bruise. This magnet was an alternating energy pattern. The next morning she had a perfect bulls-eye pattern over her bruise! Most people report warmth and gentle tingling under the magnets. Europeans have measured increased blood flow. Others have seen this on thermograms. In one month, the wound completely healed. On the basis of this case, further investigation of magnet therapy for wound healing appears to be warranted.

—*National Library of Medicine*—*J.K. Szor and R. Topp*

Magnets affect some chemical processes within and between cells. Chemists use sensitive magnetic equipment to measure simple and complex molecules.

Studies

The Effectiveness of a Magnetized Water Oral Irrigator on Plaque, Calculus and Gingival Health

The purpose of this study was to evaluate the effects of magnetized water oral irrigation on plaque, calculus and gingival health. Twenty-nine patients completed this double blind crossover study. Each patient was brought to baseline via an oral prophylaxis with a plaque index greater or equal to one and gingival index less than or equal to one.

Subjects used the irrigator for a period of three months with the magnet and three months without the magnet. After each three-month interval, data were collected using the plaque index, gingival index, and accretions indices.

The repeated measures analysis on plaque, gingival and calculus indices yielded a statistically significant period effect for the plaque index equaled .0343, the gingival index equaled .0091, and approached significance for calculus equaled .0593.

This meant that the effect of irrigation resulted in a decrease of all indices over time.

Therefore, the treatment effect on each index was evaluated using only the measurements obtained at the end of the first period (i.e., assuming a parallel design). Irrigation with magnetized water resulted in 64% less calculus compared to the control group. The reduction was statistically significant (p< or = 0.02). The reduction by 27% in gingival index was not statistically significant. The reduction in plaque was minimal (2.2 percent). A strong positive correlation between the plaque index and the Watt accretion index was observed. The magnetized water oral irrigator could be a useful adjunct in the prevention of calculus accumulation in periodontal patients but appears to have minimal effect on plaque reduction. The results indicated a clinical improvement in the gingival index, but this was not a statistically significant finding.

—National Library of Medicine—K.E. Johnson, J.J. Sanders, R.G. Gellin, and Y.Y. Palesch

Successful Treatment of an Acute Exacerbation of Multiple Sclerosis by External Magnetic Fields

A 55-year-old woman with multiple sclerosis presented with a five-week history of an exacerbation of symptoms. Prominent among these symptoms was trigeminal neuralgia, migraine headaches, blurring of vision, and ataxia of gait. While treatment with carbamazepine (Tegreto1R) (800mg/d) and oral prednisolone (15 mg/d) over a four-week period produced improvement in symptoms, externally applied magnetic fields (MF) (7.5 picoTesla; 5 HZ) placed over the scalp for a seven-minute period on three different days resulted in a complete resolution of symptoms within two weeks of initiation of treatment. Partial relief of the neuralgic pain and headaches was obtained immediately after completion of the first treatment, indicating that resolution of symptoms was related to the effects of MF and not to a spontaneous remission. This is the first report demonstrating the clinical efficacy of pico Tesla range MF in rapidly resolving an acute relapse of multiple sclerosis.

—National Library of Medicine—R Sandy and Derpapas